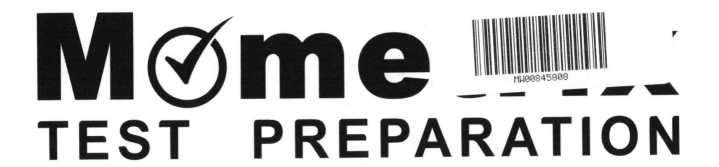

MLS
Exam Secrets
Study Guide
Part 2 of 2

DEAR FUTURE EXAM SUCCESS STORY

First of all, **THANK YOU** for purchasing Mometrix study materials!

Second, congratulations! You are one of the few determined test-takers who are committed to doing whatever it takes to excel on your exam. **You have come to the right place.** We developed these study materials with one goal in mind: to deliver you the information you need in a format that's concise and easy to use.

In addition to optimizing your guide for the content of the test, we've outlined our recommended steps for breaking down the preparation process into small, attainable goals so you can make sure you stay on track.

We've also analyzed the entire test-taking process, identifying the most common pitfalls and showing how you can overcome them and be ready for any curveball the test throws you.

Standardized testing is one of the biggest obstacles on your road to success, which only increases the importance of doing well in the high-pressure, high-stakes environment of test day. Your results on this test could have a significant impact on your future, and this guide provides the information and practical advice to help you achieve your full potential on test day.

Your success is our success

We would love to hear from you! If you would like to share the story of your exam success or if you have any questions or comments in regard to our products, please contact us at **800-673-8175** or **support@mometrix.com**.

Thanks again for your business and we wish you continued success!

Sincerely,
The Mometrix Test Preparation Team

Need more help? Check out our flashcards at:
http://mometrixflashcards.com/MLS

---

ii

TABLE OF CONTENTS

iv

Immunology

IMMUNOLOGY AND SEROLOGY TERMINOLOGY

Thermostable	Unaffected by heat.
Thermolabile	Easily affected by heat.
Physiologic	Related to body functions.
Inactivation	Destruction of biological activity, such as by heat or other agent.
Complement	A group of blood proteins that go through a cascade of interactions as part of immune response.
Reagin	Complement-fixing antibody, IgE immunoglobulin that attaches to tissue cells in the species it derives from and interacts with antigen to cause release of histamine and other vasoactive amines.
Amboceptor	Old term for hemolysin.
Hemolysin	Antibody that binds to red blood cells and lyses them to release hemoglobin.
Cardiolipin	Phospholipid that increases with some disorders, such as autoimmune and coagulation disorders.
Monoclonal	Referring to a single clone; derived from a single cell.
Polyclonal	Referring to multiple clones; derived from multiple cells.

HLA SYSTEM

HLA stands for human leukocyte antigen. The human leukocyte antigens are part of the major histocompatibility complex (MHC), a region found on chromosome 6. HLAs are found in all nucleated cells in the body. HLAs are inherited from one's parents and are practically unique to a particular individual. There are four main types of human leukocyte antigens, HLA-A, HLA-B, HLA-C, and HLA-D. Human leukocyte antigens help encode proteins on the surfaces of nucleated cells, and they play an important role in helping the body distinguish its own cells from foreign cells. Therefore, HLAs are very important when it comes to human organ transplant rejection or acceptance. In the laboratory, HLA-A, HLA-B, and HLA-C antigens can be identified using blood serum, however, HLA-D antigens can only be identified by the use of a mixed lymphocyte culture.

IMMUNOGEN, ANTIGEN, HAPTEN, ADJUVANT, AND ANTIBODY

- Immunogen: Any substance that produces an immune response
- Antigen: Any substance that reacts with substances in the immune system; antigens do not always produce an immune response
- Hapten: A molecule with a low molecular weight, which combines with another molecule to produce an antibody response
- Adjuvant: A substance that magnifies immune responses
- Antibody: A protein that fixes itself to an antigen; also known as immunoglobulins, and divided into five classes: IgA, IgD, IgE, IgG, and IgM

CLASSES OF ANTIBODIES

Every antibody has two heavy polypeptide chains and two light polypeptide chains. The identity of the heavy chains depends on the class of antibody. The light chains will be either kappa or lambda chains. Each polypeptide chain has a variable region, which identifies the particular antibody, and one or more constant regions. All of the chains are joined by disulfide bonds.

1

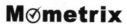

Testing and Disease States

PROGESTERONE AND HUMAN CHORIONIC GONADOTROPIN

Progesterone is a steroid hormone that is necessary to successfully maintain a pregnancy. After a woman ovulates, the level of progesterone in her blood increases dramatically. The progesterone helps prepare the uterine wall for a fertilized egg to implant, in the case of a pregnancy. The high levels of progesterone also help prevent an early spontaneous miscarriage of the pregnancy. During pregnancy, the main source of progesterone is the placenta. Progesterone also helps in the production of milk in the woman's mammary glands.

Human Chorionic Gonadotropin (hCG) is a protein hormone that is released by the placenta. hCG is released very soon after conception during a pregnancy, and it is the hormone that is often tested for with a home pregnancy test to determine the existence of a pregnancy. The level of hCG in a woman's blood is at its highest level during the first trimester of pregnancy. It drops off after that, so that a woman in her seventh month may test negative for pregnancy.

CHRONIC GRANULOMATOUS DISEASE

Chronic granulomatous disease (CGD) is a hereditary, X-linked disease in which phagocytes cannot kill pathogens. Mostly boys under 10 years old are affected, and will likely die by the age of 30. Phagocytes cannot produce superoxide anions to destroy invaders because they lack NADPH oxidase. Therefore, a patient with chronic granulomatous disease has recurrent fungal and bacterial infections, which can be fatal. This lack of NADPH enzyme also allows for oxidative products, such as hydrogen peroxide, to build up and cause death. In the laboratory, the nitroblue tetrazolium test can be used to determine the existence of chronic granulomatous disease. Patients with CGD will have neutrophils with greatly reduced nitroblue tetrazolium activity.

AUTOIMMUNE DISEASE

Any condition in which a person creates antibodies for their own antigens is an autoimmune disease. There are a couple of different theories that seek to explain autoimmune disease. The immunologic deficiency theory asserts that all of the antibodies produced by B lymphocytes are suppressed by T lymphocytes, and so antibodies are produced any time there is a decrease in T lymphocyte activity. The forbidden-clone theory asserts that occasionally lymphocytes erroneously fail to destroy autoantigens during fetal development. The theory of sequestered antigens asserts that some antigens can remain invisible to the immune system until tissue is damaged.

TYPE I HYPERSENSITIVITY

An immediate hypersensitivity is referred to as a type I hypersensitivity. This is simply an allergic reaction that occurs within minutes of contact with the allergen or antigen. An individual experiencing such a reaction is producing an increased level of IgE immunoglobulin. There are a few different laboratory tests that can be used to determine allergies by measuring total serum IgE: ELISA, RIST, RIA, and RAST.

FEBRILE AGGLUTINATION TESTS

Febrile agglutinins are antibodies that are active at normal body temperature and can cause their antigens (such as RBCs, proteins) to clump when exposed to each other, resulting in a fever. Febrile agglutinins are present in some disorders, such as systemic lupus erythematosus, hemolytic anemia, inflammatory bowel disease, and lymphoma. They may also occur in response to some infections (salmonella, brucellosis, typhoid fever) and when taking some medications (penicillin, methyldopa), so these medications may interfere with test results. To identify an infection, a blood sample is taken when a patient is actively infected (with fever and symptoms) or during

2

convalescence, diluted (20-40 times), and mixed with antigens of a specific infectious microorganism. This sample is then examined to determine if an antigen-antibody reaction has occurred. Increased IgM usually indicates a new infection and increased IgG indicates a chronic infection or history of infection.

C-REACTIVE PROTEIN AGGLUTINATION SLIDE TESTS

C-reactive protein (CRP) agglutination slide tests can be used to screen patients for CRP (qualitative test) or to determine the titer (quantitative test). A number of different test kits are available, so procedures may vary.

Qualitative test	Quantitative test
Add latex solution to positive and negative controls and serum (or diluted and undiluted serum), mix, and agitate for 2 minutes to observe for agglutination (clumping) in serum, a reaction indicating the presence of C-reactive protein.	Mix serum samples to different dilutions in saline and conduct test similar to qualitative method to determine the highest dilution that shows agglutination (positive reaction).

ANTISTREPTOLYSIN SCREEN AND TITER

Antistreptolysin O screen and titer (ASO) identifies the presence of streptolysin O antibodies, which form in response to the streptolysin O enzyme (antigen) secreted by group A β-hemolytic streptococci. The antibodies are present within one week and peak at 2-3 weeks after onset of streptococcal infection. Increased titer is present with strep-associated rheumatic fever, scarlet fever, endocarditis, and glomerulonephritis.

RHEUMATOID ARTHRITIS (RA) TESTS

Rheumatoid factor (RF)	Normal value 0-20 IU/mL. Assesses for macroglobulin type antibody that is present in connective tissue disease. Non-specific for RA
Anti-citrullinated protein antibody (ACPA)	Normal values: Negative: <20. Weakly positive: 20-39. Moderately positive: 40-59. Strongly positive: >60. Assesses for autoantibodies against citrullinated proteins, to which those with RA react.
Erythrocyte sedimentation rate (ESR)	Normal values: Age <50: 0-15 mm/h males and 0-25 mm/h females. Age >50: 0-20 mm/h males and 0-30 mm/h females. Inflammation causes increased globulins or fibrinogens, and these cause RBCs to clump and fall to the bottom of a vertical test tube. ESR is nonspecific for RA, but increased ESR may indicate increased inflammation.
C-reactive protein (CRP)	Normal value <1 mg/dL. Assesses for abnormal glycoproteins, which are produced by the liver when inflammation is present. CRP is non-specific for RA.

3

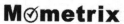

POLYCLONAL HYPERGAMMAGLOBULINEMIA AND MONOCLONAL HYPERGAMMAGLOBULINEMIA

Polyclonal hypergammaglobulinemia: A broad spike in the gamma region of the protein electrophoresis performed on a serum; indicates elevated levels of specific antibodies; the result of infectious disease, liver disease, or inflammation

Monoclonal hypergammaglobulinemia: A narrow peak in the gamma region of a protein electrophoresis performed on a serum; due to malignant transformation of a B lymphocyte clone; the results of multiple myeloma, immunoglobulin heavy chain diseases, or Waldenström's macroglobulinemia

MICROHEMAGGLUTINATION TEST FOR TREPONEMA PALLIDUM

The **microhemagglutination test for *Treponema pallidum* (MHA-TP)**, a gram-negative spirochete, is a nontreponemal antibody tests that assesses serum for antibodies to syphilis although this particular test has been generally replaced by other tests that are more specific, such as fluorescent treponemal antibody absorption (FTA-ABS), immunoassays, and molecular testing. MHA-TP can be used to confirm a positive diagnosis of syphilis on other tests. MHA-TP is able to detect antibodies to *T. pallidum* and is used for all stages of syphilis except during the first month of infection. One of the problems with MHA-TP is that false positives may occur in the presence of other infections, so it is not specific to syphilis: mononucleosis, Lyme disease, malaria, relapsing fever, leptospirosis, and leprosy. Patients with systemic lupus erythematosus may also have a false-positive on the test.

IMMUNOFLUORESCENCE REACTIONS

Direct immunofluorescence: Reagent antibody labeled with fluorescent dye reacts to a specific antigen, forming an antigen-antibody complex, and thereby suggesting the existence of a particular antigen

Indirect immunofluorescence: Unlabeled antibody reacts with antigens and a sample, forming an antigen-antibody complex; at this point, the antigen-antibody complex reacts with another labeled antibody, forming an antibody-antigen-antibody complex

Biotin-avidin immunofluorescence: A form of indirect immunofluorescence in which a labeled antibody and a labeled fluorochrome react with an antigen

TERMS RELATED TO TRANSPLANT IMMUNOLOGY

- Allograft: Tissue is transplanted from one place to another on the same individual
- Isograft: Tissue from one individual is transplanted onto a genetically identical individual
- Autograft: tissue from one individual is transplanted onto an individual from the same species
- Graft acceptance: The condition in which healing and revascularization signal the acceptance of a tissue graft or transplant
- Hyperacute graft rejection: Rejection of a graft or transplant in the first 24 hours
- Acute graft rejection: Rejection of a graft or transplant within weeks
- Chronic graft rejection: Rejection of a graft or transplant within months or years

STAGES OF INFECTION OF *TREPONEMA PALLIDUM*

Treponema pallidum infections are transmitted via sexual contact or from mother to baby in utero and are responsible for causing syphilis. **Primary** syphilis infections occur 10–90 days following exposure as painless sores at the site of inoculation. The lesions, known as chancres, are most

4

frequently located in the mouth, anus, or on the genitals and resolve on their own 3–6 weeks after they appear. Primary infections can easily be cured; however, if they are not treated, they will progress to a secondary stage. In 4–12 weeks following the resolution of the chancres, the following symptoms of **secondary** syphilis occur: a diffuse rash spreading over the entire body, generalized lymphadenopathy, patchy hair loss, and fatigue. Secondary syphilis requires treatment to eradicate the disease; otherwise, symptoms will resolve and the disease will progress to the latent stage. **Latent** syphilis is defined by patients with serologic proof of infection who do not exhibit any signs or symptoms of disease. Syphilis may remain latent for the entirety of a patient's life, or it may return years to decades after the initial infection. **Tertiary** or late-stage syphilis is characterized by immense neurological, cardiovascular, and ocular damage that may lead to death.

STAGES OF INFECTION OF *BORRELIA BURGDORFERI*

Borrelia burgdorferi is transmitted to humans via a bite from deer ticks (*Ixodes scapularis*) or mouse ticks and causes Lyme disease. Lyme disease progresses through three stages of disease, beginning with erythema migrans, which presents at the site of the tick bite as a red, ring-shaped lesion with a central clearing, reminiscent of a bullseye. Headache, muscle and joint pain, fever, malaise, and lesions on sites other than the site of inoculation also occur during the first stage of the disease. In the weeks to months following the infection, symptoms include arthritis and neurological disorders due to bacterial spread to other tissues and organs. Infections of the meninges, spinal cord, peripheral nerves, and brain are common during this second stage of Lyme disease. The final stage of disease caused by *B. burgdorferi* includes chronic arthritis and a diffuse skin rash, known as acrodermatitis chronic atrophicans, that may last for many years following an infection.

LATENT TUBERCULOSIS INFECTION

Methods used to detect latent TB infections are based on the body's development of delayed hypersensitivity and cell-mediated immune responses to antigenic components of *Mycobacterium tuberculosis* organisms. The **purified protein derivative tuberculin skin test** is performed by intracutaneously injecting culture material of *M. tuberculosis* into the forearm and visually inspecting the injection site 48–72 hours after inoculation for a firm, red bump or induration. The diameter of the induration is indicative of a patient's TB status and is interpreted as follows:

- **<5 mm**: negative
- **5–9 mm**: positive in patients with human immunodeficiency virus, recent contact with a TB-infected individual, organ transplant patients, or other immunocompromised individuals
- **10–14 mm**: positive in patients from areas with a high prevalence of TB, mycobacteriology laboratory personnel, children <4 years old, or other high-risk individuals
- **≥15 mm**: positive

Interferon gamma release, or QuantiFERON, **assays** are the gold standard for diagnosing a latent TB infection or TB disease. Whole blood samples are mixed with synthetic *M. tuberculosis* peptides and are incubated for 16–24 hours. ELISA assesses the body's response to multiple *M. tuberculosis* antigens by measuring the amount of interferon gamma released from sensitized lymphocytes. Results ≥25% of antigenic activity are considered positive for TB infection.

CYTOKINE TESTING

Cytokines are substances secreted by cells that act as mediators in the cell-to-cell connection between the innate and adaptive immune systems. **Interleukins**, **interferons**, and **growth factors** are cytokines whose expressions are highly regulated and react in response to the presence of foreign antigenic materials in the body. Cytokine testing is helpful in determining and understanding the cause of chronic or infectious inflammatory diseases because certain cytokine concentrations increase during these conditions. Single cytokines can be detected using simple **ELISA** or **chemiluminescent** assays specific to the cytokine in question. Multiple cytokines, or a panel of cytokines, can be assessed by performing a **bead-based multiplex immunoassay** methodology. The multiplex methodology uses multiple-color-coated latex beads labeled with cytokine-specific antibodies. The patient sample and the color-coated beads are added to a sample well, in which any cytokines present will bind to their complementary bead and any other biologic material is washed away. Cytokines are qualitatively and quantitatively detected by the observance and separation of the colored beads via flow cytometry.

TARGET AMPLIFICATION

Target amplification methodologies use an enzyme-mediated process to synthesize copies of a target nucleic acid sequence for the detection of infectious materials. Target amplification can be achieved via various methodologies, but all methods are based on the use of two oligonucleotide primers for target sequence detection and reproduction of in vivo replication processes. These methods provide the ability to produce between 10^8 and 10^9 copies of the target sequence for detection. The following techniques use target amplification mechanisms for the detection of infectious agent genetic materials:

- Polymerase chain reaction (PCR)
- Ligase chain reaction
- Transcription-mediated amplification
- Rolling cycle amplification
- Strand displacement amplification
- Nucleic acid sequence-based amplification

NUCLEIC ACID SEQUENCING

Nucleic acid sequence-based amplification (NASBA) testing is a non-polymerase chain reaction (PCR) target amplification methodology used for the direct detection of ribonucleic acid (RNA) viruses, including human immunodeficiency virus and hepatitis C virus. NASBA methods are specific to the amplification of RNA and ribosomal RNA even in the presence of deoxyribonucleic acid (DNA) material. In isothermal conditions, NASBA uses two target-specific oligonucleotide primers to hybridize target RNA and reproduce the replication process. The NASBA procedure and method of detection are described as follows:

1. **Primer 1** hybridizes to the target RNA sequence.
1. **Reverse transcriptase** elongates the primer's RNA copies to create a DNA/RNA hybrid.
2. **RNase H** hydrolyzes the RNA portion, leaving a single-stranded DNA molecule.
3. **Primer 2** anneals to the DNA.
4. **Reverse transcriptase** elongates primer 2, creating an active promoter site for transcription to occur.
5. **RNA polymerase** produces multiple copies of RNA transcripts that are antisense to the original target sequence.

Target sequence RNA is detected in real time by molecular beacon probes containing oligonucleotide sequences complementary to the target sequence. The hybridization of the molecular beacons to the amplified target sequence produces a fluorescence that is detected by its intensity and is directly proportional to the concentration of target RNA in a sample.

Microbiology

Preanalytic Procedures

SPECIMEN LABELING AND COLLECTION

For the best chance to recover and identify the causative organism for an infection, microbiology specimens should be collected before antibiotics are administered and collected from the site where the suspected infection is located. In addition to two patient identifiers (name, date of birth, or medical record number), the source, or where the sample was collected, should be noted on the specimen label. Specimen collection procedures vary depending on the source, but all microbiology samples must be collected into sterile containers to prevent contamination. To avoid contamination from normal flora, alcohol wipes or iodine may be used to disinfect the area above or around the source of microbiology specimens.

COMMON TRANSPORT SYSTEMS AND CONDITIONS REQUIRED FOR SPECIMENS

There are a variety of disposable culture containers that are ideal for microbiological specimen transport. Sterile swab systems with a plastic shaft are ideal for the safe transport of aerobic and anaerobic samples. Anaerobic swab systems contain gel in the bottom of the tube to support the viability of any anaerobic organisms that are present. If transport to the laboratory is delayed for more than 2 hours, most microbiology specimens can be refrigerated at 4–6 °C for temporary storage. Genital cultures and **CSF** samples should never be refrigerated, and they require immediate culturing because they are susceptible to degradation at low temperatures and contain **fastidious** organisms requiring special handling conditions. Urine, feces, and sputum may be refrigerated because the cool temperatures will help prevent the overgrowth of normal flora present in the samples.

PRIORITIZATION, REJECTION CRITERIA, BIOSAFETY CABINETS, AND PPE

All microbiology specimens should be collected prior to antibiotic administration for the best chances of cultivating pathogenic organisms for identification. Blood culture samples must be collected from two different sites to confirm septicemia and avoid false diagnosis due to contamination. Genital and CSF samples targeted for gonococcal organisms must be cultured immediately due to their fastidious nature.

Samples submitted in inappropriate collection containers or transport media meet the criteria for rejection. Anaerobic cultures cannot be set up from aerobic swab collection systems due to the exposure to air inhibiting the growth of these organisms. Any sample with leaks or risk of outside contamination cannot be accepted for culture due to the risk of false identification of organisms that have infiltrated a sterile container.

Lab coats and gloves are always necessary PPE when handling biological specimens, and biosafety cabinets provide additional protection from aerosol-inducing specimens. Sputum samples and other respiratory specimens must be handled under biosafety hoods due to the risk of aerosols being introduced into the air. These cabinets provide additional protection to eyes and the respiratory tract of lab personnel, with a glass shield and mechanisms that direct airflow up and into the hood instead of out toward lab staff.

SAMPLE PREPARATION AND MEDIA TYPES

Samples are added to various types of media to aid in the growth and identification of pathogenic organisms present in a sample. Inoculating the appropriate media related to the source of the specimen and knowledge of organisms' growth requirements are imperative to providing accurate information for patient diagnosis and treatment.

Categories of media and examples are given as follows:

- **Supportive**: contain nutrients that allow most nonfastidious organisms to grow based on their metabolism
  - **Sheep blood agar** — an all-purpose, general medium used for primary inoculations and subculturing
- **Selective:** contains dyes, antibiotics, and other compounds that inhibit some bacteria, effectively allowing others to grow
  - **Colistin plus nalidixic acid** — selective for Gram-positive, inhibits growth of Gram-negative organisms
  - **MacConkey agar and eosin methylene blue agar** — selective for Gram-negative, inhibits Gram-positive growth
- **Enrichment:** allow for the growth of one bacterium by providing nutrients specific to that organism
  - **Chocolate** — contains X and V growth factors, ideal for fastidious organisms
  - **Selenite** — favors *Shigella* and *Salmonella*
- **Differential:** contain factors that give particular organisms distinct, recognizable features
  - **Sheep blood agar and colistin plus nalidixic acid** — differentiation of organisms by hemolytic properties
  - **MacConkey agar and eosin methylene blue agar** — differentiation of Gram-negative organisms by their ability/inability to ferment lactose.

INOCULATION TECHNIQUES AND OBJECTIVES

To inoculate for **colony counts**, a sterile 10 μL loop is placed into a sample, and then it is struck down the middle of the plate in a straight line. The loop is then dragged left and right over the center line for the entire area of the plate. This allows for a standard of quantification of colonies growing on media and a clue as to how strong of an infection is present.

Inoculating media for **isolation** consists of transferring inoculum from a sterile pipette or loop and streaking it into quadrants on a plate with the goal of successively fewer colonies in each quadrant. This is achieved by heavily placing a small amount of specimen inoculum on one edge of a plate and using a loop to streak the inoculum over the first quarter or quadrant of the media. With a quarter turn of the plate, streak from quadrant one into the second quadrant, and repeat for the third and fourth quadrants. This allows for colonies to grow isolated from one another in the third and/or fourth quadrant of the plate, providing the ability to obtain pure samples of bacteria for further testing and identification.

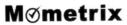

INCUBATION CONDITIONS

Common incubation and bacterial growth requirements are as follows:

Temperature	Oxygen (O_2)	Other Atmosphere
Psychrophiles Thrive in cold temperatures. Optimal temperature: 15 °C.	Aerobes require the presence of O_2 to grow.	Microaerophiles prefer lower amounts of O_2 than is present in "normal" or room air.
Mesophiles The most pathogenic organisms, which thrive at moderate temperatures, such as the human body temperature of 37 °C.	Facultative anaerobes are able to grow with or without O_2 present.	Capnophiles prefer a higher CO_2 content than regular air provides.
Thermophiles grow best in heat with optimal temperatures between 50 and 60 °C.	Obligate anaerobes are harmed by the presence of O_2 and require O_2-free environments to grow.	Aerotolerant organisms do not require the presence of O_2 to grow, but they are not harmed if O_2 is present.

SLIDE PREPARATION USING STAINS

Techniques used for microbiology slide preparation are determined by the type of sample submitted. Commonly used techniques are described below:

- **Fluid/Liquid**: Using a sterile pipette, place one drop of body fluid or other liquid samples onto the slide and swirl or spread it into a thin layer.
- **Swabs**: Roll the swab directly onto the surface of a slide. If two swabs are submitted, use one to inoculate the media and the second for slide preparation. If only one swab is submitted, inoculate all media first and roll the swab onto the slide last to avoid contamination of the media.
- **Organism colony**: Slide preparation for organism colonies requires a drop of sterile water or saline to first be added to the slide. Place the colony on the slide and mix it with the water to create a suspension.

A circle may be drawn with a wax pencil around the sample to aid in identifying where to examine on the slide. Allow the sample to air dry. Once the sample dries, slides will need to be fixed to keep the specimens from washing off during the staining process. One minute of heat fixing or the same duration fixing with 95% methanol is appropriate.

GRAM STAIN

The Gram stain is a differential stain that separates bacteria into two groups based on their reaction to the primary stain and the counterstain. This stain works by targeting the cell wall of bacteria and how they differ. The cell wall of Gram-positive organisms is made of a peptidoglycan layer with teichoic acid crosslinks, whereas the cell wall of Gram-negative organisms is comprised of a thinner peptidoglycan layer and additional outer membranes.

The Gram stain procedure consists of four elements that produce a differentiation in bacteria present on a slide. Crystal violet is used as the primary stain that stains every organism equally. Gram's iodine is then added to form a complex with the crystal violet within Gram-positive bacteria cell walls. An alcohol/acetone decolorizer then flushes away the purple color from the Gram-negative bacteria. Finally, a counterstain of safranin is introduced to stain the colorless Gram-negative organisms and allows them to be observed.

9

PROCEDURE AND INTERPRETATION OF GRAM STAIN

Gram stain procedure:

1. Flood the slide with crystal violet for 10 seconds*.
2. Rinse the slide with water.
3. Flood the slide with Gram's iodine for 10 seconds*.
4. Rinse with water.
5. Quickly add decolorizer until the slide runs clear (no color) for ~10 seconds.
6. Rinse with water.
7. Flood the slide with safranin for 10 seconds*.
8. Rinse with water.
9. Allow the slide to air dry.
10. Examine under an oil immersion lens.

*Time increments may vary; 30- or 60-second intervals are common as well.

Outcome:

- Gram-positive bacteria will stain purple/blue.
- Gram-negative bacteria will stain pink.

Along with the color of the bacteria, the shape and morphology are able to be determined with a Gram stain. Information provided from this stain is helpful in determining subsequent tests, culture, and means for identification. It may also guide treatment because some antibiotics work better toward Gram-positive or Gram-negative organisms specifically.

ACID-FAST STAIN

The acid-fast stain, also called the **Ziehl–Neelsen** stain, is performed to detect organisms that cause tuberculosis. These bacteria are deemed acid-fast bacilli (**AFB**) due to their ability to be visualized by the acid-fast staining process. This is a differential stain for mycobacterium that will retain the primary stain, whereas all other bacteria, without a cell wall containing mycolic acid, will decolorize and counterstain.

The acid-fast procedure consists of the primary stain, carbolfuchsin, with heat to facilitate penetration of the stain into the cell walls of mycobacterium with high lipid content. A 3% hydrochloric acid, 97% ETOH decolorizer is then used to leach the primary stain from the cell walls of bacteria that do not contain high contents of mycolic acid. Methylene blue is used as a counterstain to make all of the other bacteria a visible blue color.

Acid-fast/Ziehl–Neelsen procedure:

1. Heat fix stain/slide for 2 hours at 65–70 °C or 15 minutes at 80 °C.
2. Flood stain with heated carbolfuchsin at 60 °C for 5 minutes.
3. Rinse with water.
4. Decolorize with 3% HCl/97% ETOH ~2 minutes (for an average-thickness slide).
5. Rinse with water.
6. Flood with methylene blue 1–3 minutes.
7. Rinse with water.
8. Allow to air dry.
9. Examine under an oil immersion lens.

Interpretation:

- Mycobacterium (AFB) will stain red.
- All other bacteria will stain blue.

MODIFIED ACID-FAST STAIN

The modified acid-fast stain, or **Kinyoun** stain, is performed to detect organisms that cause tuberculosis by differentiating **AFB** from all other bacteria in a microbiology specimen. This achieves the same outcome as the acid-fast stain, without the use of heat. The modification of heat requirements means that the Kinyoun stain is also referred to as "cold" acid-fast staining.

This method uses a carbolfuchsin stain prepared with phenol to facilitate the penetration of stain into the lipid-rich cell walls of mycobacteria. An acid/alcohol solution, comprised of 3% HCl and 97% ETOH, is used to decolorize nonmycobacterium organisms by removing the primary stain from their cell walls. A counterstain of methylene blue or malachite green is used to allow decolorized bacteria to become visible again upon examination, allowing for differentiation to occur.

Modified acid-fast/Kinyoun procedure:

1. Heat fix stain/slide for 2 hours at 65–70 °C or 15 minutes at 80 °C.
2. Flood stain with Kinyoun carbolfuchsin at room temperature for 5 minutes.
3. Rinse with water.
4. Decolorize with 3% HCl/97% ETOH for ~2 minutes (for an average-thickness slide).
5. Rinse with water.
6. Flood with methylene blue or malachite green for 1–3 minutes.
7. Rinse with water.
8. Allow to air dry.
9. Examine under an oil immersion lens.

Interpretation:

- Mycobacterium (AFB): red
- All other bacteria: blue (methylene blue) or green (malachite green).

POTASSIUM HYDROXIDE (KOH) REAGENT

Potassium hydroxide (**KOH**) reagent is used to aid in the direct examination of yeast and fungal elements present in samples, including, but not limited to, vaginal discharge, skin, hair, and nails. Presence of fungal elements upon visualization aids in the diagnosis and treatment process of suspected fungal infections.

The 10–20% KOH reagent that is added to specimens clears debris and breaks down keratin in hair and nail samples. The breakdown of keratin and the clearing of other debris allows for fungal elements to be more readily observed with a light microscope on a clean glass slide.

KOH procedure:

1. Place the specimen on a clean glass slide — use clean forceps for hair/skin/nail or roll a swab with vaginal discharge/wound sample onto the slide.
2. Add one drop of KOH reagent to the sample on the slide.
3. Place a glass coverslip over the area of the slide; press gently to reduce the presence of bubbles.

4. Place the slide on the microscope stage and examine on low (10×) power to visualize the presence of any fungal structures, such as hyphae or budding yeast.
5. If fungal structures are observed, examine the slide at 40× magnification for further identification and verification of fungi.

CALCOFLUOR-WHITE STAIN

Calcofluor-white is a nonspecific chemifluorescent stain that binds to the cellulose and chitin in cell walls of fungal and parasitic organisms, allowing for visualization via a fluorescent microscope. KOH may be added to the white stain to clear the sample of debris and allow for better visualization. With this method, chitin-containing structures will fluoresce white on a dark background with ultraviolet (UV) light. Evans blue is used as a counterstain to create a dark field, and it allows cells and tissues to be fluoresced and visualized under blue light. Fungal and parasitic elements will fluoresce a bright apple-green color, and all of the other elements will fluoresce at a red-orange color for differentiation between them.

Calcofluor-white procedure:

1. Place the specimen on a clean glass slide.
2. Add one drop of calcofluor-white stain and one drop of KOH (optional) to the slide.
3. Place a glass coverslip over the slide, and press gently to reduce the presence of bubbles.
4. Let the specimen stain, and stain for 1 minute.
5. Examine under UV light at 100× to 400× magnification for the presence of yeast, fungi, or parasitic elements.

TRICHROME STAIN

The trichrome stain is a permanent stain that allows for visualization of and morphological distinguishing of parasitic cysts and trophozoites in clinical specimens. The most common specimens submitted for trichrome staining are fresh or preserved stool fecal samples; however, other clinical specimens are able to be stained with polyvinyl alcohol (PVA) fixation.

The trichrome stain consists of chromotrope 2R, light green SF, phosphotungstic acid, glacial acetic acid, and distilled water. Stain preparation is necessary, by adding 1 ml of acetic acid to the dry components, allowing the mixture to stand for 30 minutes, and then adding 100 ml of distilled water. The stain should be purple in color and should be protected from light. Proper fixation of slides is included in the trichrome procedure because it is necessary for quality staining and optimal use of this method.

Trichrome procedure:

1. Prepare a fresh fecal smear or PVA smear.
2. Place the slide in 70% ETOH for 5 minutes — for PVA smears, skip this step.
3. Remove the slide and drain off the excess liquid.
4. Place the slide in 70% ETOH with added iodine (dark reddish-brown color) for 2–5 minutes.
5. Remove the slide and drain off the excess liquid.
6. Place the slide in 70% ETOH for 5 minutes.
7. Remove the slide and drain off the excess liquid.
8. Place the slide in clean/new 70% ETOH for 2–5 minutes.
9. Remove the slide and drain off the excess liquid.
10. Place the slide in a prepared trichrome stain solution for 10 minutes.
11. Remove the slide and drain off the excess stain.
12. Dip the slide in 90% ETOH acidified with 1% acetic acid up to 3 seconds (no longer).

13. Dip once in 100% ETOH.
14. Place the slide in 100% ETOH for 2–5 minutes.
15. Place the slide in clean/new 100% ETOH for 2–5 minutes.
16. Place the slide in xylene for 2–5 minutes.
17. Repeat the slide in xylene for 2–5 minutes.
18. Mount the slide with a cover glass, and allow it to dry overnight at 37 °C.
19. Observe with a fluorescent microscope.

Outcome:

- Background debris — green
- Protozoa — blue-green to purple; the nuclei and inclusions of parasites will show red to purple-red.

GIEMSA STAIN

Giemsa stain is used in the visualization, differentiation, and identification of parasites in clinical specimens. Most commonly, Giemsa stains are performed on blood smears, but they may be performed on specimens from other sources as well, such as lesion biopsies and various aspirates. Thin-film smears allow for RBC inclusion and extracellular morphologies to be more easily observed, whereas thick smears allow a larger volume of sample to be surveyed for potential parasites. Giemsa-stained blood films are used as diagnostic testing for malarial infections, due to the *Babesia* parasite present demonstrating the characteristic "Maltese cross" ring formation.

Prepared from a powder containing azure, methylene blue, eosin dye, and methanol, Giemsa stock stain is diluted with buffered water to properly stain slides for observation. In blood smears, the Giemsa stain color in parasites will mimic the color of the stained WBCs. This acts as an internal quality control for the method. The morphologic characteristics of parasites observed with this stain are used for differentiation and subsequent identification.

Giemsa stain procedure:

1. Place a slide into absolute methanol for 30 seconds to fix a thin sample to the slide. (Skip this step for thick slides; methanol fixation is not needed.)
2. Allow the slide to air dry.
3. Place the slide in 1 part Giemsa stock stain to 20 parts buffered water for 20 minutes*.
4. Remove the slide and drain off the excess stain.
5. Dip the slide in buffered water one to two times to wash the slide.
6. Remove the slide and allow it to air dry, propped in a vertical position.
7. Observe the slide under a 40× lens and then under an immersion lens with a light microscope.

*Dilutions of Giemsa stock stain may vary between 10 and 50, depending on the preparation. The staining time must be adjusted for the different stain concentration present. Typically, the dilution factor will correspond to the appropriate duration of staining (e.g., 1:10, 10 minutes; 1:30, 30 minutes).

Outcome:

- Parasitic forms: blue to purple with reddish nuclei
- RBCs: pale gray-blue
- WBC nucleus, cytoplasm: purple, pale-purple, respectively

- Eosinophilic granules: bright purple-red
- Neutrophilic granules: deep pink-purple.

ACRIDINE ORANGE

Fluorochrome acridine orange is a nonspecific stain that binds to nucleic acids. This stain is used to confirm the presence of bacteria in blood culture smears in the following instances: the Gram stain is difficult to interpret, the presence of bacteria is highly suspected but not observed via light microscopy, or for the detection of bacteria incapable of retaining Gram stains, such as mycoplasmas.

Acridine Orange Procedure:

1. Fix a blood culture smear to a glass slide with heat or methanol.
2. Flood the slide with acridine orange, allowing the stain to remain on the slide for two minutes without drying.
3. Rinse the slide with tap water and allow to air dry.
4. Examine under ultraviolet fluorescent microscopy.

Interpretation:

Any bacteria or host cells present will fluoresce bright orange against a dark or green-fluorescing background.

Analytic Procedures—Bacteriology

BLOOD AND BONE MARROW
SPECIMEN SOURCES AND COLLECTION TO CHECK FOR INFECTION IN BLOODSTREAM

To diagnose an infection in the bloodstream, or **sepsis**, the most common samples collected are blood cultures. **Blood cultures** consist of blood being added to aerobic and anerobic bottles containing a broth that supports microbial growth. Ideally, two sets of blood cultures will be collected from separate sites to compare results and more easily determine false positives due to contamination from true-positive results. If infection originating from a port or intravenous catheter is suspected, draw one set of cultures from the port or catheter line and the other set peripherally. Intravenous catheter tips may cause infection from opportunistic skin flora at the time of insertion or removal of the device. After removal, the catheter tip itself may be cultured if it is a suspected source of infection.

The procedure for peripheral collection of blood cultures is as follows:

1. At the site chosen to draw, aseptically cleanse the skin in a circular motion with 70% alcohol, and allow it to dry.
2. Repeat cleansing of the site with iodine, allow it to dry for 1 minute.
3. Following proper phlebotomy practices, insert the needle into the vein and withdraw the blood. Do not change the needle before injecting the blood into the blood culture bottle. The necessary volume for blood culture bottles to achieve a 1:10 dilution of blood to broth is 10 mL for adult aerobic or anaerobic and 5 mL for pediatric patients.
4. Repeat the procedure at a second draw site.

14

CONTINUOUS BLOOD CULTURE MONITORING SYSTEMS

Blood culture monitoring systems continuously assess blood culture bottles for the presence of bacterial growth. Cultures are incubated at 35–37 °C for 5–7 days in a chamber that is constantly rocking to promote the growth of any potential pathogens that are present. Gas sensors in the chamber use fluorescence to detect any CO_2 production within the blood culture bottles. The CO_2 gas production, turbidity, lysis of RBCs, and visual observation of bacterial colonies in a blood culture bottle are indicative of bacterial growth. If bacterial growth is detected, the system will alarm to notify lab staff that the presumptively positive blood culture bottle should be subcultured and Gram stained for organism detection and identification.

Continuous monitoring systems are advantageous because they monitor bacterial growth without the need to visually inspect bottles each day or blindly subculture and Gram stain every blood culture collected. Monitoring systems can also be interfaced with laboratory information systems (LIS) to allow for easier reporting of results and for reducing the risk of clerical errors.

RAPID IDENTIFICATION AND ANTIBIOTIC RESISTANCE DETECTION OF MICROORGANISMS

Rapid identification of microbial agents and their relationship to antibiotics allows for patient treatments to begin more quickly and aids in finding the most effective means to fight against an infection. Organisms can be evaluated for specific **biochemical reactions** that can aid in the presumptive identification of an infectious agent. The following biochemical tests are used in differentiating bacteria from one another: catalase, coagulase, oxidase, indole, L-pyrrolidonyl-β-naphthylamide (PYR), urease, motility, and results of various stains. **Automated instrumentation** allows for microdilutions of an isolate to be identified and evaluated for antibiotic susceptibility or resistance. An inoculum of a pure colony grown from culture media is added to sterile water or saline to create a 0.5 McFarland standard. The inoculum is added to panels of microwells with a specific reaction taking place in each well. Automated instruments are able to produce quantitative results for antibiotic susceptibility and resistance in 3–8 hours, along with a definitive identification of the organism. **Molecular techniques** are available for the rapid detection of antibiotic-resistant organisms, such as methicillin-resistant *Staphylococcus aureus* (MRSA), vancomycin-resistant *Enterococcus* (VRE), extended-spectrum beta-lactamases (ESBLs), and carbapenem-resistant *Enterobacteriaceae* (CRE). Molecular methods are able to detect the presence or absence of a gene that is specific to the antibiotic resistance; for example, PCR methods are used to detect and amplify the mecA gene responsible for MRSA strains.

SKIN FLORA

The skin's normal flora is comprised of organisms that inhabit the skin and are routinely **commensal**, meaning they don't cause harm to a healthy host. Although skin flora can be beneficial, they can also become pathogens under certain circumstances by displacement to another part of the body or **opportunistic** infection in an immunocompromised host. Species of skin flora inhabit different areas of the body based on the environment that part of the body produces. Common skin flora grow in the axilla, perineum, toe webs, hands, face, trunk, and upper arms and legs.

Skin flora commonly include the following organisms:

- **S. aureus** — colonizes in the nasal passages, most common to become pathogenic
- **Staphylococcus epidermidis** — most prevalent skin flora, attach to the outer layer of skin, the epidermis, and inhibit overgrowth of potential pathogens
- **Corynebacterium** (diphtheroid) and **Propionibacterium acnes** — typically found in the sebaceous glands.

15

S. AUREUS AND COAGULASE-NEGATIVE STAPHYLOCOCCI

S. aureus react and present in the following ways:

- Biochemical reactions:

Catalase	+
Coagulase	+

- **Gram stain**: Gram-positive cocci in "grape-like" clusters
- **Growth requirements**: aerobic and facultative anaerobe, grows= best at 35 °C in ambient air or a CO_2-rich environment
- **Colony morphology**: soft, opaque or pale gold, and circular on sheep blood agar, most colonies are beta-hemolytic, and colonies present with a yellow halo on mannitol salt agar

Coagulase-negative *Staphylococci* react and present in the following ways:

- Biochemical reactions:

Catalase	+
Coagulase	−

- **Gram stain**: Gram-positive cocci in clusters
- **Growth requirements**: aerobic and facultative anaerobe, grow best at 35 °C in ambient air or a CO_2-rich environment
- Colony morphology:
  - ○ **S. epidermidis** — white, cohesive, raised circular colonies on tryptic soy agar, opaque, gray, smooth, raised colonies with no hemolysis on sheep blood agar
  - ○ **S. saprophyticus** — white-yellow, opaque, smooth, raised colonies with a butter-like texture on sheep blood agar.

BETA-HEMOLYTIC STREPTOCOCCI

Beta-hemolytic *Streptococci* react and present in the following ways:

- Biochemical reactions:

Catalase	−
Gas production	−
Motility	−
Optochin	R
Bile solubility	−
Leucine aminopeptidase	+
Vancomycin	S

- **Gram stain:** Gram-positive cocci in chains
- **Growth requirements:** 5–10% CO_2 with vertical stabs in agar to promote beta-hemolysis
- **Colony morphology:** the groups of beta-hemolytic strep present on sheep blood agar as follows:
  - ○ **Group A** — grayish-white, transparent to translucent, matte or glossy, large zone of hemolysis

- o **Group B** — larger than group A colonies, translucent to opaque, flat, glossy, narrow zone of beta-hemolysis, and some strains are nonhemolytic
- o **Group C** — grayish-white, glistening, wide zone of beta-hemolysis
- o **Group F** — grayish-white, small, matte, narrow zone of beta-hemolysis
- o **Group G** — grayish-white, matte, wide zone of beta-hemolysis.

ENTEROCOCCUS SPECIES

Enterococcus species react and present in the following ways:

- Biochemical reactions:

Catalase	−
PYR	+
Gas production	+
Optochin	R
Bile solubility	−
Bile esculin	+
6.5% NaCl	+
Leucine aminopeptidase	+

- **Gram stain:** Gram-positive cocci in chains or diplococci
- **Growth requirements:** aerobic and facultative anaerobe, able to grow in temperatures ranging between 10 °C and 45 °C
- **Colony morphology:** large white colonies on sheep blood agar, may be alpha- or beta-hemolytic, blackens medium of bile esculin agar during growth.

CANDIDA SPECIES

Candida species present in the following ways:

- **Gram stain**: Gram-positive single yeast buds, pseudohyphae constricted but connected at the ends, or true septate hyphae
- **Growth requirements**: aerobic and facultative anaerobe, grow best at 25–37 °C
- **Colony morphology**: creamy, white, dull, grows upward with foot-like projections from the bottom of the colony on sheep blood agar and cream-colored, smooth, pasty colonies on Sabouraud dextrose agar.

STREPTOCOCCUS PNEUMONIAE

Streptococcus pneumoniae react and present in the following ways:

- Biochemical reactions:

Catalase	−
Bacitracin	R
Na Hippurate	−
Optochin	S
Bile solubility	+
Bile esculin	−
6.5% NaCl	−

- **Gram stain**: Gram-positive diplococci, lancet shaped
- **Growth requirements**: facultative anaerobe, grow best at 35–37 °C in a 5% CO_2 environment
- **Colony morphology**: alpha-hemolytic, mucoid or "water drop" colonies with a convex middle on sheep blood agar.

ACINETOBACTER BAUMANNII

Acinetobacter baumannii react and present in the following ways:

- Biochemical reactions:

Oxidase	–
Growth on MacConkey agar	+
Motile	–
Glucose oxidation	+
Maltose oxidation	–
Esculin hydrolysis	–
Lysine decarboxylase	–
Nitrate reduction	–
Urea	V

- **Gram stain**: Gram-positive/variable coccobacilli
- **Growth requirements**: aerobic and facultative anaerobe, grow best at 35 °C in ambient air or a CO_2-rich environment
- **Colony morphology**: smooth, creamy, opaque, raised on sheep blood agar, purplish hue on MacConkey agar.

ENTEROBACTERIACEAE

Enterobacteriaceae react and present in the following ways:

- Biochemical reactions:

Oxidase	–
Catalase	+
Nitrate reduction	+

- **Gram stain**: Gram-negative bacilli
- **Growth requirements**: aerobic and facultative anaerobe, grow best at 35 °C in ambient air or a CO_2-rich environment. MacConkey and other selective agars are incubated in ambient air only. *Yersinia pestis* grow best at 25–30 °C.
- **Colony morphology**: large, smooth, and gray on sheep blood and chocolate agars.
  - o Lactose fermenting species, pink on MacConkey agar:
    - ❖ Citrobacter
    - ❖ Escherichia
    - ❖ Enterobacter
    - ❖ Klebsiella

- Lactose nonfermenting species, colorless to pale on MacConkey agar:
  - ❖ Shigella
  - ❖ Yersinia
  - ❖ Proteus
  - ❖ Salmonella

PSEUDOMONAS SPECIES

Pseudomonas species react and present in the following ways:

- Biochemical reactions:

Motility	+
Oxidase	+
Indole	+
Lysine decarboxylase	−

- **Gram stain**: Gram-negative bacilli
- **Growth requirements**: obligate aerobe, grow best at 35 °C in ambient air or a CO_2-rich environment
- **Colony morphology**:
  - ***P. aeruginosa*** — grayish white, translucent to opaque, circular with irregular edges on sheep blood agar. Colorless, transparent, circular, on MacConkey agar. Colonies are smooth or mucoid, if swarming occurs. Produce a grape, or corn tortilla-like odor.

BACTERIA COMMONLY RESPONSIBLE FOR INFECTIVE ENDOCARDITIS

Infective endocarditis results in inflammation and damage to heart valves and the inner lining of the heart, the **endocardium**. Endocarditis occurs when bacteria are introduced to the bloodstream and settle in this portion of the heart, creating acute or subacute infections. **Acute** infections typically cause great damage to a healthy heart and require more aggressive treatment, whereas **subacute** infections are less virulent and generally attack weaker hearts with preexisting conditions.

The following bacteria are common agents of endocarditis:

- *Staphylococcus aureus:*
  - Most common cause of acute endocarditis — damage to a healthy heart
  - Normal skin flora introduced through broken skin barrier
    - ❖ Intravenous drug abuse
    - ❖ Infected abscess
    - ❖ Contamination during surgery or catheterization procedures
- *Streptococcus viridans:*
  - Most common cause of subacute endocarditis — damage to a weak heart with congenital heart defects
  - Normal oral flora introduced by a breach in the oral mucosa
    - ❖ Dental procedures
    - ❖ Poor oral hygiene
- *S. epidermidis* (coagulase-negative *Staphylococci*):
  - Most associated with infections of prosthetic heart valves

- o Normal skin flora introduced through broken skin barrier
  - ❖ Cardiac catheterization procedures
  - o Often requires surgical intervention to treat
- *Enterococcus* and *Streptococcus bovis*:
  - o Subacute, nosocomial infections
  - o Normal GI/genitourinary flora introduced via exacerbated infection or malignancy.

AGENTS OF BONE MARROW INFECTION

An infection of the bone and bone marrow is known as osteomyelitis. **Osteomyelitis** occurs when bacteria are introduced to the bone tissue in the following manners: as an extension of a local soft-tissue, urogenital, or respiratory-tract injury; carried via the bloodstream; surgery; an open fracture; or intravenous drug use. The most common causative agent of osteomyelitis in all patients is *Staphylococcus aureus* because it resides in the body and on the skin as normal flora and is pathogenic when traumatically introduced into other tissues and the bloodstream.

Salmonella **species** are the most common organism to cause osteomyelitis in patients with sickle cell disease. *Salmonella* osteomyelitis typically involves the diaphysis, or shaft, of the long bones in children. *Brucella* **species** are zoonotic organisms that can infect humans via ingesting undercooked meat or unpasteurized dairy, inhaling the bacteria, or traumatic entrance through the skin and mucous membranes via injury. Brucellosis presents as an acute febrile illness and may be misdiagnosed, leading to the spread of disease to the bone.

Osteomyelitis caused by the group B strep species, *S. agalactiae*, is seen in newborns who acquire an infection from their mother during birth. Newborns and children may develop bone marrow infections from the manifestation of infections caused by group A strep, *Streptococcus pyogenes.*

VIRULENCE MECHANISMS

Although *Brucella* **species** organisms are not encapsulated, they possess an antigenic lipopolysaccharide outer surface. O-antigens on the surface of the organism allow for the bacteria to invade and enter host cells for replication and survival. Complement does not easily bind to *Brucella* surface lipopolysaccharides, providing the bacteria the ability to evade host immune responses and proliferate. Another key virulence factor for *Brucella* species is the organism's ability to survive extreme temperatures and pH levels, allowing it to thrive in various parts of the body and allowing infections to spread.

Sickle cell disease patients affected by *Salmonella* **species** infections are extremely susceptible to sepsis and osteomyelitis infections caused by these organisms. Fimbriae and H antigens on the outer surface of the bacteria aid in its adherence to cells in the host's body. Surface proteins and antigens, including antiphagocytic proteins, capsular antigens, H flagellate antigens, and immunogenic O antigens, prevent phagocytosis and complement-mediated lysis of bacterial cells. Lipid A in the outer layer of *Salmonella* species organisms is released upon the death of the bacterial cell and is the endotoxin responsible for the fever and shock associated with these infections.

The virulence of *S. aureus* begins with the organism's rigid peptidoglycan cell wall and surface capsular antigens, which inhibit phagocytosis and promote adherence to host cells. Teichoic acids in the cytoplasmic membrane and cell wall of *S. aureus* promote adhesion, colonization, and bacterial cell division in hosts. Protein A facilitates biofilm formation and adhesion, and it binds to receptors on host immunoglobulins allowing *S. aureus* to evade phagocytosis. Fibronectin-binding proteins present in methicillin-resistant bacteria strains also promote the formation of a biofilm, which is described as a thin, slimy film of bacteria that adheres to the surface of host cells and tissues. Cellular toxicity and destruction of host cells is achieved by red blood cell toxic hemolysins, white blood cell toxic leukocidin, and heat-stable enterotoxins. Enzymes produced by *S. aureus* also aid in the virulence of the bacteria in the human body by degrading the host's response to an infection, facilitating the spread of disease.

S. agalactiae also contains a rigid cell wall with polysaccharide capsular antigens that inhibit complement activation and prevent phagocytosis. This **group B streptococcus** species produces C5a peptidase, a protein that deters complement and neutrophil chemotaxis, and participates in adhesion and invasion of host cells. Pore-forming hemolysin toxins promote organism entry into host cells and facilitate its survival. *S. agalactiae* organisms resist intracellular phagocytosis and spread infection by the actions of the following cell surface proteins: C antigen, cell surface penicillin-binding protein, and hyaluronidase.

CEREBROSPINAL FLUID (CSF)

CSF COLLECTION

A **lumbar puncture** procedure consists of a needle being inserted through a patient's back between two lower vertebrae and moved into the space surrounding the spinal cord. The space surrounding the spinal cord is filled with cerebrospinal fluid (CSF) that will drip from the needle once properly inserted. Fluid will then be collected into sterile containers for laboratory testing.

CSF collection from a **ventricular shunt** is accomplished through the placement of a catheter behind the ear that will drain excess spinal fluid from the brain. A shunt is inserted into the ventricles of the brain to relieve pressure caused by an accumulation of CSF. Catheter tubing is placed to divert excess CSF either outside of the body for sterile collection or to other parts of the body, such as the pleural or peritoneal cavities, to be absorbed by blood vessels.

A catheter may be placed into a lateral ventricle that is attached to a **reservoir** implanted under the scalp for external access to a shunt system. The reservoir is often used to deliver drugs directly to the CSF and CNS or to aspirate CSF for testing with a syringe in a minimally invasive manner.

HAEMOPHILUS INFLUENZAE

Haemophilus influenzae react and present in the following ways:

- **Biochemical reactions**:

Catalase	+
Oxidase	+
X factor (hemin)	+
V factor (NAD)	+
Beta-hemolytic on sheep blood agar	−
Lactose fermentation	−
Mannose fermentation	−

- **Gram stain:** Gram-negative bacilli
- **Growth requirements:** aerobic and facultative anaerobe, grow best on chocolate agar in 5–10% CO_2 at 35–37 °C
- **Colony morphology:**
  - **Unencapsulated strains** — small, smooth, and translucent on chocolate agar
  - **Encapsulated strains** — larger, mucoid, with a mouse nest odor on chocolate agar.

NEISSERIA MENINGITIDIS

Neisseria meningitidis react and present in the following ways:

- **Biochemical reactions**:

Catalase	+
Oxidase	+
Nitrate reduction	−
Maltose fermentation	+
Glucose fermentation	+
Lactose fermentation	−

- **Gram stain:** Gram-negative diplococci
- **Growth requirements**: aerobic and facultative anaerobe, grow best in a humid, 5–10% CO_2 environment at 35–37 °C
- **Colony morphology:** a green hue may be present on agar underneath colonies
  - **Unencapsulated strains** — medium, round, smooth, gray to white, moist on chocolate and sheep blood agar
  - **Encapsulated strains** — more mucoid appearing.

ESCHERICHIA COLI

Escherichia coli react and present in the following ways:

- **Biochemical reactions**:

Indole	+
Citrate	−
Hydrogen sulfide (H_2S)	−
Lysine decarboxylase (LDC)	+
Lysine deaminase (LDA)	−
Urease	−
Motility	+
Voges–Proskauer	+
Triple sugar iron (TSI) agar	A/A
Gas production	+

- **Gram stain**: Gram-negative bacilli
- **Growth requirements**: aerobic and facultative anaerobe, grow best at 37 °C
- **Colony morphology**: circular, convex colonies, dull gray, smooth on sheep blood agar, pink to red, surrounded by dark-pink precipitate on MacConkey agar, and yellow on Hektoen and xylose lysine deoxycholate agar (XLD) agars.

LISTERIA MONOCYTOGENES

Listeria monocytogenes react and present in the following ways:

- **Biochemical reactions**:

Catalase	+
Motility at 20–25 °C	+
Esculin	+
Nitrate reduction	−
Christie–Atkins–Munch–Petersen (CAMP) test	+
Hippurate	+
Glucose fermentation	+

- **Gram stain:** Gram-negative bacilli or coccobacilli
- **Growth requirements:** aerobic and facultative anaerobe, grow best at 35–37 °C in ambient air or 5–10% CO_2
- **Colony morphology:** white, translucent, smooth, moist, with a narrow zone of beta-hemolysis on sheep blood agar.

CORYNEBACTERIUM AND PROPIONIBACTERIUM SPECIES

Corynebacterium species react and present in the following ways:

- **Biochemical reactions**:

Catalase	+
Motility	−
Esculin	−
Mycolic acids	+

- **Gram stain:** Gram-positive bacilli, slightly curved, with rounded ends — some species are pleomorphic, presenting a Chinese letter formation appearance
- **Growth requirements:** aerobic and facultative anaerobe, grow best at 35–37 °C in ambient air or 5–10% CO_2
- **Colony morphology**: on sheep blood agar
  - ○ ***Corynebacterium diphtheriae*:** varying morphology from small, gray, and translucent to medium, white, and opaque; black or gray colonies on cystine-tellurite blood agar
  - ○ **Less virulent *Corynebacterium* species:** small to medium, gray, white, or yellow, nonhemolytic colonies

Propionibacterium species react and present in the following ways:

- **Gram stain:** Gram-positive bacilli, pleomorphic, diphtheroid-like, may be club shaped or in palisade arrangements
- **Growth requirements**: anaerobic, grow best at 35–37 °C for 48 hours
- **Colony morphology:** small white to gray on anaerobic blood agar. More mature colonies will be larger and yellow colored.

CORRELATION OF CSF CULTURE AND GRAM STAIN RESULTS WITH OTHER TEST RESULTS IN DIAGNOSIS OF MENINGITIS

Correlating the appearance, microbiology, cell count, and chemistry testing of a CSF sample will provide evidence for determining the presence of a meningitis infection, as well as differentiate the causative agent. The expected results of a **normal CSF** sample free of infection are as follows:

- Appearance: clear and colorless
- Protein: 15–45 mg/dL
- Glucose: 60–70% plasma glucose levels
- Cell count: 0–5 WBC/µL
- Differential: 70% lymphocytes, 30% monocytes.

Abnormalities in the color and clarity of a CSF sample can be indicative of the following: a traumatic tap; current, recent, or previous subarachnoid hemorrhage; and infection. Evidence of a **traumatic tap** will show blood in collection tubes, with a successive clearing in each tube, a clear supernatant when spun, and clots from the presence of fibrinogen. Samples will contain blood in every collection tube during a current **subarachnoid hemorrhage**, appear pale-pink to pale-orange in a recent hemorrhage, and appear yellow in a past hemorrhage. A cloudy sample, maybe due to increased WBCs, can be indicative of an infection.

Bacterial infections can be detected and a presumptive causative organism can be seen on a Gram stain of CSF and correlated with the cell count and chemistry results.

The correlating CSF results and their etiology are as follows:

Etiology	CSF Protein	CSF Glucose	WBC Population	Lactate
Bacterial	Greatly increased	Decreased	Neutrophils	Increased
Viral	Increased	Normal	Lymphocytes	Normal
Fungal	Increased	Normal to decreased	Lymphocytes Monocytes	Increased

DIRECT AND MOLECULAR METHODS USED IN DETECTION OF CSF INFECTIONS

Direct detection methods for the evaluation and diagnosis of CSF infections includes stains, rapid latex antigen testing, and serological testing. Bacterial meningitis can be detected by the presence of bacteria found on a Gram stain. India ink and acid-fast stain preparations allow for the direct detection of *Cryptococcus* and tuberculosis pathogens, respectively. Rapid latex antigen tests are useful in the immediate detection of classic meningitis causing bacteria such as *S. pneumoniae, H. influenzae,* group B strep, *E. coli, Neisseria meningitides,* and *Cryptococcus neoformans.* Latex beads coated with sensitized monoclonal IgG antibodies for each bacterium are added to a test card with a CSF sample, mixed, and mechanically rotated for 5 minutes. Agglutination of the latex determines the presence of bacterial antigens, thus indicating a bacterial infection. Serological methods are also used in determining syphilis infections of the CNS. The fluorescent treponemal antibody absorption test is very sensitive but less specific in CSF samples than serum. Molecular methods aid in detecting pathogens that do not grow on routine media or in patients who have already had antibiotic treatments. PCR testing is available for the detection and amplification of nucleic acids in the RNA or DNA of various CSF pathogens including bacteria, virus, fungi, and parasites.

COMMON MENINGITIS-CAUSING PATHOGENS

Bacterial meningitis is caused by opportunistic bacteria that enter the bloodstream, are carried across the blood–brain barrier to the meninges, and spread throughout the spinal fluid. The etiology, transmission, and virulence of common meningitis-causing bacteria are listed below:

S. pneumoniae, H. influenzae, and **N. meningitidis** are normal flora of the upper respiratory tract and are spread from person to person by respiratory droplets. The most susceptible population are children younger than 5 years of age, and pneumonia or bacteremia are commonly the initial infection in a host prior to meningitis.

- *S. pneumoniae*
  - Pneumolysin: antiphagocytic capsular protein
  - Several adhesion factors and immunogenic cell wall membrane
- *H. influenzae* and *N. meningitidis*
  - Encapsulated strains: resistant to phagocytosis and complement-mediated lysis
  - *H. influenzae*: B strain, most likely to cause meningitis
  - *N. meningitidis*: most common meningitis causing strains: A, B, C, Y, W.

E. coli and **L. monocytogenes** are transmitted via the ingestion of contaminated food. Along with **Streptococcus agalactiae**, they are common pathogens of neonatal meningitis due to transmission from mother to baby at birth.

- *S. agalactiae* (group B strep)
  - Polysaccharide capsule: prevents phagocytosis
  - Pore-forming toxins: promote entry into host cells and facilitate organism survival
- *E. coli*
  - K1 strain: inhibits phagocytosis and resists bactericidal activity of serum antibodies
- *L. monocytogenes*
  - Escape phagocytic vacuoles due to listeriolysin O, phospholipase A, and phospholipase B.

COMMON PATHOGENS OF CSF SHUNT INFECTIONS

The following are normal skin flora organisms that act as opportunistic pathogens when introduced into the CNS at the shunt surgical site, in the shunt itself, or in the CSF fluid. Contamination of the shunt can occur during surgery to implant the device or during the aftercare and maintenance of the shunt. Virulence factors are as follows:

- Coagulase-negative *Staphylococcus*
  - Encapsulated serotypes: resistant to phagocytosis
  - Several adhesion factors and biofilm producing the cell wall membrane
- *Corynebacterium*
  - Toxigenic strains are lysogenic due to exotoxin production
- *Propionibacterium*
  - Acquired resistance to the following antibiotic classes:
    - ❖ Macrolides: erythromycin and azithromycin
    - ❖ Lincosamides: clindamycin
    - ❖ Tetracyclines: doxycycline and minocycline.

25

BODY FLUIDS FROM NORMALLY STERILE SITES

SOURCES AND COLLECTION OF SPECIMENS FOR BODY FLUIDS OF NORMALLY STERILE SITES

Sterile fluids in several cavities of the body are necessary for protection and normal function of the organs they surround. During disease or infection, these fluids can accumulate and become harmful. Collection of these fluids for analysis requires an aseptic surgical needle puncture into a membrane or cavity where fluid is then aspirated and placed into sterile collection containers. The following are sources of normally sterile fluids able to be collected for analysis:

- **Serous fluids** surround the pericardial, pleural, and peritoneal cavities.
  - ○ **Pericardial** fluid exists in the space surrounding the heart.
  - ○ **Pleural** fluid is present around the lungs in the thoracic cavity.
  - ○ **Peritoneal** fluid, or **ascites,** resides in the abdominal and pelvic cavities.
- **Synovial fluids** surround and lubricate the joints in the body.
- **Vitreous** liquid fills the space between the lens and retina of the eye, whereas the **aqueous humor** fills the anterior and posterior chambers of the eye.
- **Amniotic fluid** surrounds the fetus in the uterus during pregnancy.

INDIGENOUS ORGANISMS ASSOCIATED WITH SKIN AND MUCOSAL SURFACES

The mucous membrane is composed of layers of tissue that line the cavities in the body and cover the surfaces of internal organs. Mucosal surfaces and their associated indigenous organisms function together to protect exogenous pathogens from entering the body. Colonization of commensal normal flora inhibits the growth of potential pathogens by competing for nutrients on the surface of mucous membranes. Most indigenous species have a commensal or mutualistic relationship with the mucous membrane by coexisting or equally benefiting from one another. The following mucosal surfaces are home to the associated organisms:

- **Skin** — *S. aureus, S. epidermidis, Corynebacterium,* and *Propionibacterium acnes*
- **Conjunctiva (eyes)** — *S. aureus, S. epidermidis, S. pneumoniae, H. influenzae, Neisseria species, Candida, Aspergillus,* and *Penicillium*
- **Oral cavity and nasal passages** — *S. aureus, S. epidermidis, S. pneumoniae, S. pyogenes, S. mitis, S. salivarius, S. mutans, Enterococcus faecalis, H. influenzae, Neisseria species, E. coli, Proteus, Corynebacterium, Lactobacillus, Actinomycetes, Candida, Mycoplasmas,* and *Cryptococcus*
- **Lower respiratory tract** — *Staphylococcus, Streptococcus, Fusobacterium, Acinetobacter, Pseudomonas, Sphingomonas, Prevotella, Megasphaera, Candida,* and *Aspergillus* species
- **Gastrointestinal tract** — *Lactobacillus, Clostridium, Bacteroides, Enterococcus, Streptococcus, Corynebacterium, Enterobacter,* and *Helicobacter* species
- **Genitourinary tract (vaginal)** — *Lactobacillus, S. aureus, S. epidermidis, E. faecalis, S. pneumoniae, S. pyogenes, Neisseria species, E. coli, Proteus species,* and *Corynebacterium.*

NEISSERIA AND ACINETOBACTER SPECIES

Neisseria species react and present in the following ways:

- **Biochemical reactions**:

Catalase	+
Oxidase	+
Nitrate reduction	+

- **Gram stain:** Gram-negative diplococci
- **Growth requirements**: aerobic and facultative anaerobe, grow best in a humid, 5–10% CO_2 environment at 35–37 °C
- **Colony morphology:** small, white to gray-brown, smooth, butter-like, and translucent on sheep blood agar with a green hue on agar underneath colonies possible

Acinetobacter species react and present in the following ways:

- **Biochemical reactions**:

Oxidase	−
Catalase	+
Motile	−
Nitrate reduction	−

- **Gram stain**: Gram-negative coccobacilli
- **Growth requirements**: aerobic and facultative anaerobe, grows best at 35 °C in ambient air or a CO_2-rich environment
- **Colony morphology**: smooth, round, mucoid, opaque to white colonies on sheep blood agar.

PSEUDOMONAS AERUGINOSA

Pseudomonas aeruginosa react and present in the following ways:

- **Biochemical reactions**:

Motility	+
Oxidase	+
Catalase	+
Urease	−
Indole	−
Methyl red	−
Voges–Proskauer	−
Tryptic soy agar	K/K

- **Gram stain**: Gram-negative bacilli
- **Growth requirements**: obligate aerobe, grow best at 35 °C in ambient air or a CO_2-rich environment
- **Colony morphology**: grayish white, translucent to opaque, circular with irregular edges on sheep blood agar. Colorless, transparent, circular on MacConkey agar. Colonies are smooth or mucoid, if swarming occurs. Produces a grape, or corn tortilla-like odor.

CLOSTRIDIUM PERFRINGENS

Clostridium perfringens react and present in the following ways:

- **Biochemical reactions**:

Indole	–
Urease	–
Lecithinase	+
Nagler test	+
Reverse CAMP test	+
Vancomycin	S
Kanamycin	S
Colistin	R

- **Gram stain:** Gram-positive to Gram-variable bacilli, straight rods with blunt ends, boxcar shape. Some strains are spore forming.
- **Growth requirements:** anerobic, grow best at 35–37 °C
- **Colony morphology:** gray to grayish yellow, circular, dome-shaped, translucent, and glossy, with a double zone of beta-hemolysis on anaerobic sheep blood agar.

BACTEROIDES FRAGILIS GROUP

Bacteroides fragilis react and present in the following ways:

- **Biochemical reactions**:

Nitrate reduction	–
Urease	–
Motility	–
Growth on bile	+
Reverse CAMP test	+
Vancomycin	R
Kanamycin	R
Colistin	R

- **Gram stain:** Gram-negative bacilli, pleomorphic with rounded ends — commonly resemble a safety pin
- **Growth requirements:** anaerobic, grow best at 35–37 °C
- **Colony morphology:** convex, circular, white to gray, and translucent with no hemolysis on anaerobic sheep blood agar. At 48 hours of growth, colonies are >1 mm, circular, and gray, surrounded by a gray zone on Bacteroides bile esculin agar.

MOLECULAR TECHNIQUES TO PROCESS BODY FLUID SAMPLES

Although microscopic and culture techniques are still the main source of body fluid infection detection, molecular methods are continuing to be developed for more rapid detection of disease. PCR techniques for the detection of bacteria or fungi are available for the improved management of immunosuppressed or high-risk patients. Most available PCR techniques rely on the amplification and sequencing of the 16SrRNA gene in bacteria and the internal transcribed region 2 in fungi.

Amniotic fluid is often sent for molecular analysis for the presence of specific genetic markers linked to diseases, such as Down syndrome and cystic fibrosis, or infection, such as cytomegalovirus. PCR methods focus on the amplification of gene sequences unique to the disease being tested for.

COMMON PATHOGENS OF NORMALLY STERILE BODY FLUIDS

Infections of normally sterile body fluids occur by the introduction of bacteria to a body cavity during an invasive procedure, from a traumatic injury, or from the bloodstream. Common body fluid pathogens and their virulence factors are listed below:

- *Neisseria* species
  - Outer membrane pili: enhance adhesion and inhibit phagocytosis
  - Lipopolysaccharide endotoxin and IgA proteases
  - Encapsulated strains: resistant to phagocytosis and complement-mediated lysis
- *S. aureus*
  - Exotoxins: hemolysins, leukocidins, spreading factor by coagulase and hyaluronidase, nuclease, protease, and lipase
  - Most strains; penicillin resistance due to beta-lactamase
  - MRSA: methicillin-resistant strain
- Beta-hemolytic *streptococcus*
  - O_2-stable streptolysin S, O_2-labile streptolysin O
  - Streptococcal pyrogenic exotoxin B: inhibits action of immunoglobulins, cytokines, and complement
  - Hyaluronidase acts as a bacterial spreading factor
- *Enterococcus*
  - Adhesion factors facilitating binding to host cells, inducing cell and tissue destruction
  - Intrinsic antibiotic resistance of various species:
    - ❖ Beta-lactam antibiotics: penicillin, cephalosporin, carbapenem
    - ❖ Aminoglycosides: vancomycin-resistant *Enterococcus* (VRE)
- *Enterobacteriaceae*
  - All species release lipopolysaccharide endotoxin; some also produce exotoxins
  - H, K, and O antigens
  - Some strains express resistance to carbapenem antibiotics
- *P. aeruginosa*
  - Lipopolysaccharide endotoxin, hemolysins, protease
  - Exotoxin A: toxic to macrophages, prevents phagocytosis
  - Encapsulated: inhibits phagocytosis and actions of complement
- *C. perfringens*
  - *C. perfringens* enterotoxin, alpha and beta toxins: damage tissues, blood vessels, and blood cells
  - Hemolysins, proteases, lipases, collagenase, and hyaluronidase: aid in invasive processes
- *B. fragilis*
  - Polysaccharide encapsulation: protects from phagocytosis, stimulates abscess formation
  - Penicillin resistance due to beta-lactamase

LOWER RESPIRATORY
SOURCES AND COLLECTION OF LOWER RESPIRATORY TRACT SAMPLES

Lower respiratory tract specimens can be collected from the sources and with the methods described below.

Ideal **sputum** specimen collection occurs first thing in the morning, with no food ingestion for 1–2 hours prior. Rinsing the mouth with water before collection and collecting directly into a sterile specimen container aid in avoiding contaminating the sample with saliva. Sputum is collected through the following methods:

- **Expectorated** sputum is expelled by a deep cough by the patient.
- **Induced** sputum collection uses an aerosol spray that reaches the lungs, inducing a deep cough.
- **Endotracheal aspirate** samples are collected via mechanical suction from patients with a tracheostomy tube.

Bronchoscopy procedures visualize the lungs by passing a tube with a light source and camera down a patient's throat and into the lungs. Bronchoscopes are used for collection of the following lower respiratory tract specimens:

- **Bronchial washings** are collected from the bronchial tubes. A measured amount of sterile saline is passed through the scope, and then it is gently suctioned back out. The suctioned saline is placed into a sterile container because it contains the cells and fluids needed for analysis.
- **Bronchoalveolar lavage** samples are collected from the smaller bronchoalveolar pathways via the same process as bronchial washings. Multiple lavage samples may be collected from several sites during one procedure.
- **Bronchial brushings** are collected by passing a brush through the bronchoscope and gently abrading the surface of the airway mucosa and bronchial lesions to collect cells for analysis.

QUANTITATIVE AND SEMIQUANTITATIVE RESULT REPORTING OF LOWER RESPIRATORY TRACT SPECIMENS

Quantitative and semiquantitative results from Gram stains of lower respiratory tract specimens are used to evaluate the quality of samples before culture and aid in the diagnostic and treatment process for patients suspected of lower respiratory tract infections. Expectorated and induced sputum samples must meet specific Gram stain criteria to be considered acceptable for culture. Observed in 10–20 fields under low power, the following criteria indicate an acceptable specimen: <10 squamous epithelial cells and ≥10 WBCs per field. Regardless of the number of white cells present, samples with more than 25 epithelial cells per low-power field will be rejected. These results indicate that a sample did not originate in the lower respiratory tract and is contaminated by saliva and oral flora. Gram stains of acceptable lower respiratory tract samples are examined further under the oil immersion lens. Under this lens, any bacteria present are evaluated for their Gram stain reaction and morphologic characteristics and are semiquantitatively enumerated as rare, few, moderate, or many. Physicians interpret semiquantitative results for bacteria in conjunction with quantitative WBC and epithelial cell results to determine the following: the presence or absence of infection, the presumptive cause of infection, and the severity of infection.

ORAL FLORA

The oral cavity is home to a variety of organisms whose Gram stain and colony morphology on sheep blood agar are described below:

- Gram-positive cocci:
  - *Staphylococcus*
    - ❖ *S. aureus*: soft, opaque or pale gold, and circular
    - ❖ *S. epidermidis*: opaque, gray, smooth, raised, with no hemolysis
  - *Streptococcus*
    - ❖ *S. pneumoniae*: alpha-hemolytic, convex, mucoid or "water drop"
    - ❖ *S. pyogenes*: grayish-white, transparent to translucent, matte or glossy, large zone of hemolysis
    - ❖ *S. mitis*: alpha-hemolytic, broken glass appearance
    - ❖ *S. salivarius*: small, colorless, smooth or rough, nonhemolytic or weakly alpha-hemolytic
    - ❖ *S. mutans*: small white to gray, rough, nonhemolytic or alpha-hemolytic
  - *E. faecalis*: circular, smooth, nonhemolytic
- Gram-positive bacilli:
  - *Corynebacterium*: small to medium, gray, white, or yellow, nonhemolytic
  - *Actinomycetes*: white, rough, crumbly texture, occasionally pigmented red
  - *Lactobacillus*: small to medium, gray, alpha-hemolytic
- Gram-positive buds, hyphae, or pseudohyphae:
  - *Candida*: creamy, white, dull, grows upward with foot-like projections
- Gram-negative cocci:
  - *Neisseria*: small, white to gray-brown, smooth, butter-like, translucent, possible green hue underneath
- Gram-negative bacilli:
  - *H. influenzae*: on chocolate agar
    - ❖ Unencapsulated strain — small, smooth, and translucent
    - ❖ Encapsulated strain — larger, mucoid, with a mouse nest odor
  - *E. coli*: circular, dull gray, smooth, convex.

COMMON LOWER RESPIRATORY TRACT PATHOGENS

Infections of the lower respiratory tract are caused by the following organisms whose Gram stain and colony morphology on sheep blood agar are described below:

- Gram-positive cocci:
  - *S. aureus*: soft, opaque or pale gold, and circular
  - *S. pneumoniae*: alpha-hemolytic, convex, mucoid or "water drop"
- Gram-negative bacilli:
  - *H. influenzae*: on chocolate agar
    - ❖ Unencapsulated strain — small, smooth, and translucent
    - ❖ Encapsulated strain — larger, mucoid, with a mouse nest odor
  - *K. pneumoniae*: small to medium, grayish-white, translucent or opaque. circular, dome shaped, mucoid, nonhemolytic

- ○ *Legionella*: green or iridescent pink, circular with entire edge, convex, glistening, with a ground-glass appearance on buffered charcoal yeast extract agar
- Mycoplasma pneumoniae:
  - ○ Organisms do not stain well due to the lack of a rigid cell wall.
  - ○ Pinpoint, granular, "fried egg" appearance on media enriched with cholesterol and fatty acids.
- Mycobacterium tuberculosis
  - ○ Mycolic acid in the cell wall resists Gram stain. Appear as slim rods, gram variable or bright red using an acid-fast stain.
  - ○ Off-white to buff, dry, rough, raised, and wrinkled on Löwenstein–Jensen medium.
- Fungi
  - ○ Yeasts: Gram-positive buds, hyphae, or pseudohyphae
    - ❖ *Candida*: creamy, white, dull, grows upward with foot-like projections
  - ○ Other fungi: fluorescent white buds, hyphae, or pseudohyphae with KOH reagent and calcofluor-white stain
    - ❖ Variable growth on Sabouraud's dextrose agar for up to 6 weeks after inoculation.

LEGIONELLA AND M. TUBERCULOSIS

Legionnaires' disease and Pontiac pneumonia are lower respiratory infections caused by **Legionella** bacteria. *Legionella* bacteria's natural habitat is freshwater lakes and ponds, and it becomes pathogenic when it is able to grow in human-made water systems such as air conditioners, shower heads, hot water heaters, and large plumbing systems. Water aerosols containing the bacteria are inhaled and can cause disease.

Legionella

- Heat shock protein 60: aids in invasion
- Outer membrane protein: prevents phagocytosis
- Type IV pili: entry into macrophages for spread and survival.

Primary infections caused by **M. tuberculosis** take place in the lungs causing pneumonia-like symptoms. If left untreated, tuberculosis can become disseminated and spread to other organ systems in the body.

M. tuberculosis

- No endotoxins or exotoxins, toxic effects on cells from lipids and phosphatides
- Cord factor: destroys cell mitochondria, inhibits leukocyte migration
- Waxy layer and mycolic acid cell wall: delay hypersensitivity, induce multidrug-resistant variants.

Opportunistic fungi such as **Aspergillus** and **Cryptococcus** species aspirated into the lungs can cause pneumonia and lead to sepsis in immunocompromised patients. Bacterial lung abscesses are commonly a polymicrobial infection predominantly comprised of **anaerobic oropharyngeal or gastric normal flora** aspirated into the lungs.

DIRECT AND MOLECULAR TECHNIQUES FOR DETECTING RESPIRATORY PATHOGENS

S. pyogenes, or group A *Streptococcus,* is the respiratory pathogen responsible for upper respiratory infections including strep throat and pharyngitis, whereas *B. pertussis* is responsible for whooping cough. These infections are very contagious, and quick, accurate detection is vital to reduce the spread of these organisms.

Rapid test kits have been created for the detection of *S. pyogenes* using **immunochromatographic** or **immunofluorescent assays**. Positive results are enough evidence to diagnose infection, whereas negative results need to be confirmed with a throat culture. **Direct-fluorescent antibody testing** is a serologic test for the presence of IgG antibodies to *B. pertussis.* Although helpful in diagnosing an infection of *B. pertussis,* a diagnosis will be delayed because this method is best when a patient is tested between 2 and 8 weeks of symptom onset. Traditional culture or molecular methods allow for a timelier diagnosis for *B. pertussis* than antibody testing.

The most common molecular method used to detect *S. pyogenes* and *B. pertussis* is **real-time PCR**, with specific nucleic acid probes of <200 base pairs for each organism. **Multiplex PCR** methods are also used to detect *B. pertussis,* along with multiple other respiratory pathogens. The highly specific **isothermal loop-mediated amplification** method can also be used in detecting *B. pertussis* infections between 0 and 3 weeks of symptom onset.

COMMON PNEUMONIA-CAUSING PATHOGENS

Lower respiratory tract infections can manifest into various disease states including tracheitis, acute or chronic bronchitis, and community- or hospital-acquired pneumonia. The mode of transmission for these pathogens is through the inhalation of respiratory droplets from an infected person. Common pneumonia-causing pathogens and their associated virulence are described below:

- *S. aureus*
  - Exotoxins: hemolysins, leukocidins, spreading factor by coagulase and hyaluronidase, nuclease, protease, and lipase
  - Beta-lactamase: penicillin resistance, MRSA: methicillin resistance
- *S. pneumoniae*
  - Pneumolysin: antiphagocytic capsular protein
  - Several adhesion factors and immunogenic cell wall membrane
- *H. influenzae*
  - Encapsulated strains: resistant to phagocytosis and complement-mediated lysis
- *Klebsiella pneumoniae*
  - Encapsulated to inhibit phagocytosis and complement-mediated lysis
  - Lipopolysaccharide endotoxin causing inflammation
  - Fimbriae for adhesion and siderophores that acquire host iron for organism survival
- *M. pneumoniae*
  - P1 membrane protein: acts as a cytohesin to ciliated epithelial cells
  - Community-acquired respiratory distress syndrome toxin: damages respiratory epithelium and ciliary activity by releasing cytokines and inflammatory mediators.

UPPER RESPIRATORY

UPPER RESPIRATORY TRACT SAMPLES

Upper respiratory tract samples collected with a swab require a plastic shaft flocked swab and the appropriate transport media for the potential pathogens, whether aerobic, anaerobic, or viral. Specimens collected to evaluate for such infections include the following:

- **Throat** swabs are placed in the back of the throat, and the tonsillar area is vigorously swabbed in patients suspected of strep throat infections.
- **Nasal** swab collection consists of a swab inserted at least a half inch into the nostril, firmly rotated, and left in place for 10–15 seconds. Repeat the process in the other nostril using the same swab.
- **Nasopharyngeal** swab collection requires a thin, flexible swab that is more easily inserted into the nasopharyngeal passage. The patient's head should be tilted back slightly at a 70° angle to straighten the passage from the nares to the nasopharynx. Gently insert the swab through the nose, to the posterior nares, rotate it several times, and remove.
- **Sinus** exudate samples are collected via direct needle aspirate of the sinus or with a swab during surgical procedures of the sinuses.
- **Middle ear** samples are collected with a swab or needle aspirate. If the patient's eardrum has ruptured, the fluid released into the outer ear can be collected by inserting a sterile swab into the ear using an auditory speculum. Neonates, the elderly, or patients with persistent, chronic, or recurrent otitis media may have middle ear fluid collected via tympanocentesis, requiring a sterile needle puncture through the tympanic membrane to aspirate the middle ear fluid.

MAJOR PATHOGENS OF UPPER RESPIRATORY TRACT

Infections of the upper respiratory tract are caused by the following organisms whose Gram stain and colony morphology on sheep blood agar are described below:

- Gram-positive cocci:
  - *S. pyogenes*: grayish-white, transparent to translucent, matte or glossy, large zone of hemolysis
  - *S. pneumoniae*: alpha-hemolytic, convex, mucoid or "water drop"
- Gram-positive bacilli in a "Chinese letter" formation:
  - *C. diphtheriae*: small, circular, convex, white to gray
- Gram-negative coccobacilli:
  - *B. pertussis*: small, round, shiny, silver colored, becoming whitish gray with age on charcoal blood agar
- Gram-negative bacilli:
  - *H. influenzae*: on chocolate agar
    - ❖ Unencapsulated strain — small, smooth, and translucent
    - ❖ Encapsulated strain — larger, mucoid, with a mouse nest odor
  - *P. aeruginosa*: grayish-white, translucent to opaque, circular with irregular edges

COMMON THROAT, OROPHARYNX, AND EAR PATHOGENS

Upper respiratory infections caused by **S. pyogenes, C. diphtheriae, B. pertussis,** and **H. influenzae** are transmitted by inhaling respiratory droplets of an infected individual or touching the mouth and nose with a contaminated hand or object. Throat and oropharynx pathogens' virulence factors are described below:

- *S. pyogenes*
  - O_2-stable streptolysin S, O_2-labile streptolysin O
  - Erythrogenic toxin: causes scarlet fever rash
  - Streptococcal pyrogenic exotoxin B: inhibits immunoglobulins, cytokines, and complement actions
  - M protein: prevents phagocytosis
  - Hyaluronidase: bacterial spreading factor
- *C. diphtheriae*
  - Diphtheria toxin: inhibits protein synthesis, leading to the death of host cells, and is carried in the bloodstream to other organs causing paralysis and CHF
  - Pili structures and proteins for adherence and colonization
    - SpaA, B, and C: selective to pharyngeal epithelial cells
    - SpaD and H: selective for lung and laryngeal epithelial cells
- *B. pertussis*
  - Adhesion and colonization factors
    - Filamentous hemagglutinin
    - Pertussis toxin: specific to tracheal endothelium; S2 adheres to ciliated epithelial cells and S3 adheres to phagocytes
  - Lipopolysaccharide endotoxin
  - Invasive adenylate cyclase: reduces local phagocytic activity
  - Lethal toxin: localized inflammation, issue necrosis
  - Tracheal cytotoxin: kills ciliated respiratory epithelium

Ear infections are not contagious; they manifest from upper respiratory infections. **P. aeruginosa** cause swimmer's ear, developing from moisture in or damage to the ear canal. Middle ear infections, otitis media, occur along with or following other upper respiratory symptoms caused by **S. pneumoniae** or **H. influenzae**.

GASTROINTESTINAL

SALMONELLA SPECIES

Salmonella species react and present in the following ways:

- **Biochemical reactions**:

Indole	−
Citrate	+
H$_2$S	+
LDC	+ *
LDA	−
Urease	−
Ornithine decarboxylase (ODC)	+
Motility	+
TSI agar	K/A
Gas production	Variable

*Key differentiating characteristics.

- **Gram stain**: Gram-negative bacilli
- **Growth requirements**: mainly aerobic but facultative anaerobe as well, 37 °C with growth in 16–24 hours of inoculation.
- **Colony morphology**: opaque or translucent, smooth, 2–4 mm in diameter on supportive media, green or transparent with black center on Hektoen enteric agar, transparent or red with black centers on xylose-lysine-deoxycholate agar.

SHIGELLA SPECIES

Shigella species react and present in the following ways:

- **Biochemical reactions**:

Indole	Variable
Citrate	−
H$_2$S	− *
LDC	−
LDA	− *
Urease	−
ODC	Variable
Motility	− *
TSI agar	K/A
Gas production	−

*Key differentiating characteristics.

- **Gram stain**: Gram-negative bacilli
- **Growth requirements**: aerobic and facultative anaerobe, 35 °C with growth 18–24 hours after inoculation
- **Colony morphology**: clear or slightly pink on MacConkey agar, green or transparent on Hektoen agar, transparent or red on xylose-lysine-deoxycholate agar

36

TOXIGENIC ESCHERICHIA COLI

Toxigenic *Escherichia coli* react and present in the following ways:

- **Biochemical reactions:**

Indole	+
Citrate	−
H_2S	−
LDC	+
LDA	−
Urease	−
ODC	+
Motility	+
TSI agar	A/A
Gas production	+

- **Gram stain**: Gram-negative bacilli
- **Growth requirements**: aerobic and facultative anaerobe, grow best at 37 °C
- **Colony morphology**: circular, convex colonies, gray, translucent to opaque on sheep blood agar, pink, opaque on MacConkey, green with a metallic sheen, opaque on eosin methylene blue agar.

CAMPYLOBACTER SPECIES

Campylobacter species react and present in the following ways:

- **Biochemical reactions:**

Catalase	+
Oxidase	+
Hippurate	+

- **Gram stain**: Gram-negative bacilli, small curved rods, "seagull appearance"
- **Growth requirements**: Microaerophilic, *Campylobacter*-selective agar at 42 °C
- **Colony morphology**: mucoid, flat, grayish colonies with irregular edges, potentially swarming.

Vibrio species react and present in the following ways:

- **Biochemical reactions:**

Catalase	+
Oxidase	+

- **Gram stain**: Gram-negative bacilli, curved rod with polar flagella
- **Growth requirements**: aerobic and facultative anaerobe, require media with increased salt concentration, sodium chloride, and acidic pH, 35–37 °C for 6–8 hours for APW or 35–37 °C 18–24 hours to TCBS and all other media.
- **Colony morphology**: creamy white, smooth and convex; yellow-green on TCBS, colorless on MacConkey agar.

YERSINIA ENTEROCOLITICA

Yersinia enterocolitica react and present in the following ways:

- **Biochemical reactions:**

Indole	V
Citrate	–
H$_2$S	–
LDC	–
LDA	–
Urease	V
ODC	+
Motility	V*
TSI agar	K/A
Gas production	–
Catalase	+
Oxidase	–

*Motile at 22–25 °C; nonmotile at 37 °C (body temperature).

- **Gram stain**: Gram-negative bacilli
- **Growth requirements**: aerobic and facultative anaerobe, grow optimally at room temperature (22–25 °C)
- **Colony morphology:** translucent or opaque or gray-white, slightly mucoid (after 24 hours of growth) on sheep blood agar, flat, colorless or pale pink on MacConkey agar, "bulls-eye" appearance with deep-red center and translucent outer zone on cefsulodin irgasan novobiocin (CIN) agar.

AEROMONAS SPECIES

Aeromonas species react and present in the following ways:

- **Biochemical reactions:**

Indole	+
Citrate	+
H$_2$S	V
LDC	+
Urease	–
ODC	–
Motility	V
TSI agar	K/A
Gas production	V
Catalase	+
Oxidase	+

- **Gram stain**: Gram-negative bacilli, single, in pairs, or short chains
- **Growth requirements**: aerobic and facultative anaerobe, grow best at 35–37 °C
- **Colony morphology:** circular, gray on sheep blood agar, dark green on sheep blood agar after 72 hours due to beta-hemolysis, deep-red center surrounded by translucent outer zone of colony on CIN agar.

PLESIOMONAS SHIGELLOIDES

Plesiomonas shigelloides react and present in the following ways:

- **Biochemical reactions:**

Indole	+
Citrate	
H$_2$S	
LDC	+
LDA	
Urease	
ODC	–
Motility	
TSI agar	K/A
Gas production	–
Catalase	+
Oxidase	+

- **Gram stain**: Gram-negative bacilli
- **Growth requirements**: aerobic and facultative anaerobe, grow best at 35–37 °C
- **Colony morphology:** clear and colorless on MacConkey, CIN, and XLD agars, clear and green on Hektoen agar.

DIRECT AND MOLECULAR TECHNIQUES FOR DETECTING CLOSTRIDIUM DIFFICILE- AND SHIGA TOXIN-PRODUCING ORGANISMS

Due to their ability to cause life-threatening infections, the rapid detection of *C. difficile*- and Shiga toxin-producing *E. coli* organisms is pertinent for prompt patient care. Although exclusion of these organisms is possible, current methodologies alone cannot provide a definitive diagnosis for active infections and require interpretation along with clinical and epidemiological findings.

Direct immunochromatographic *C. difficile* testing methods simultaneously target the glutamate dehydrogenase (GDH) antigen and toxins A and B produced by toxigenic strains. Similarly, rapid tests for Shiga toxins 1 and 2 use antibody-labeled assays to determine the presence or absence of toxigenic strains of *E. coli*. Evaluations of these tests are as follows:

- *C. difficile*:
  - GDH antigen and toxin absent: no *C. difficile* infection
  - Both GDH antigen and toxin present:
    - ❖ Symptomatic: consistent with active infection
    - ❖ Asymptomatic: consistent with *C. difficile* colonization
  - Either GDH antigen or toxin present: inconclusive; molecular testing recommended
- Shiga toxin (ST1 and ST2):
  - ST1 and ST2 absent: no Shiga toxin-producing *E. coli* present
  - Either ST1 or ST2 or both present: Shiga toxin-producing *E. coli* present.

PCR and nucleic acid amplification testing molecular methods provide a definitive rule-out or supportive diagnosis of toxigenic infections. Nucleic acid amplification testing targets genes specific to toxigenic *C. difficile* strains including toxins A and B and 16S ribosomal RNA. Genes for ST1, ST2,

E. coli O157:H7, and *Shigella dysenteriae* type 1 are targeted for detection of Shiga toxin-producing organisms.

SEROTYPING *E. COLI*, *SALMONELLA*, AND *SHIGELLA* ORGANISMS

Serotyping allows for the differentiation of species and subspecies of organisms that otherwise have indistinguishable physical and biochemical properties. Determining the serotype of enteric pathogens allows for further insight on disease manifestations and proper treatment methods. Serotyping can be completed using the following test methodologies: bacterial, latex, or coagglutination, and fluorescent or enzyme-labeled immunoassay.

E. coli, Salmonella, and *Shigella* species and subspecies are differentiated from one another by the antigenic properties of their O, K, and H antigens. Present in the outermost layer of the bacterial cell wall, the **O antigen** is a polymer of immunogenic repeating oligosaccharides. The **K antigen** is present in the capsular polysaccharides, and a threadlike structure portion of the flagella in motile organisms contains the **H antigen**. More than 2,000 *Salmonella* serotypes have been detected and are determined by their individual expression of the O and H antigens. Based on their O antigenic properties, *Shigella* organisms are organized into four main species, or serogroups: A (*S. dysenteriae*), B (*S. flexneri*), C (*S. boydii*), and D (*S. sonnei*), which can be further divided further into several serotypes. *E. coli* subspecies are differentiated based on the composition and immunogenic properties of the O, K, and H antigens; for example, *E. coli* O157:H7 is the extremely dangerous subspecies that produces a *Shigella*-like toxin that causes an enterohemorrhagic response.

MAJOR GASTROINTESTINAL PATHOGENS

Gastrointestinal infections occur from humans ingesting bacteria present in raw, undercooked, or unpasteurized products or human to human via the fecal–oral route. Reservoirs and virulence mechanisms of major gastrointestinal pathogens are described below:

Pathogen	Reservoir	Virulence Factors
Salmonella	Poultry	Lipopolysaccharide endotoxin: intracellular survival O and H antigens: immunogenic, motility Adhesion, colonization, and antiphagocytic properties Type III secretion system for survival in macrophages
Shigella	Human	Endotoxins: invasion, multiplication, and antiphagocytic properties Adhesion factor: colonization O antigen, Shiga toxin: immunogenic, inhibits cell protein synthesis causing life-threatening disease Type III secretion system: invading macrophages
P. shigelloides	Soil, water, seafood	Enterotoxins, invasins, and hemolysin
Aeromonas species	Amphibians, reptiles, fish; more prevalent during warm-weather months	Lophotrichous flagella: motility Various toxins, proteases, hemolysins, lipases, adhesins, and agglutinins
Y. enterocolitica	Swine	Lipopolysaccharide endotoxin Protein capsular antigen: protects against phagocytosis Proteins to promote adhesion and invasion

40

Pathogen	Reservoir	Virulence Factors
Campylobacter species	Poultry, cattle, and sheep	Lipopolysaccharide endotoxin and exotoxins Superoxide dismutase: harmful to cells' DNA or membrane factors Siderophores: iron sequestering
E. coli	Cattle	O, K, and H antigens: immunogenic, encapsulation, motility K1: inhibits phagocytosis, resists serum antibody activity O157:H7: hemorrhagic effects
Vibrio species	Water, oysters, other seafood	Adhesion factor, pili: colonization, mucosa adherence Hemagglutination protease: intestinal inflammation and degradation Cholera toxin: quickly causes severe dehydration Siderophores

DETECTION METHODS FOR HELICOBACTER PYLORI

Serological tests using monoclonal IgG *H. pylori* antibodies or polyclonal *H. pylori* antibodies can be used to **screen** for a past or present infection. Antigens produced by the presence of *H. pylori* can be detected in serum or stool samples by binding to antibodies embedded in a test cartridge and migrating to a test window where they produce a colored line. Positive results obtained by serological methods often require confirmation with another method to diagnose an *H. pylori* infection.

The **urea breath test** is a confirmatory method used for the detection of an active *H. pylori* infection or to monitor the efficacy of treatment. *H. pylori* rapidly metabolizes urea, and it is excreted as carbon molecules in the breath. For this method, patients ingest urea capsules that contain radioactively labeled carbon molecules and then they exhale into a collection container 10–15 minutes after swallowing the capsule. Breath samples are qualitatively analyzed for the presence or absence of the radioactive labeled carbon molecules. Their presence in a sample confirms an active infection in patients seeking a diagnosis and determines that the infection has not been eradicated in patients undergoing treatment.

Direct detection of *H. pylori* can be determined from gastric or duodenal biopsy specimens via microscopy, culture, or molecular methods.

Histological identification of the organism observed in Gram-stained smears or imprints of biopsy samples yields the presence of curved Gram-negative bacilli. **Culture** of these specimens is required if antibiotic susceptibility testing is needed for treatment options. Although culture methods are difficult to perform, *H. pylori* present in biopsied tissue will grow on solid, blood agar media in a microaerophilic environment.

An infection can also be confirmed by performing a **rapid urease test** by placing a biopsy specimen in agar or on a reaction strip containing urea, a buffer, and a pH indicator. Urease from *H. pylori* will metabolize the urea to ammonia and bicarbonate, increasing the pH in the test system, and change the color of the pH indicator to reflect the alkaline environment. Results can be determined in 1–24 hours and confirm the presence of an active infection.

Polymerase chain reaction (PCR) testing is highly specific and is more sensitive for *H. pylori* detection than other methods. Target sequences of bacterial DNA present are amplified, replicated, and identified if it is present in a sample.

SKIN, SOFT TISSUE, AND BONE

SKIN, SOFT-TISSUE, AND BONE CULTURES

Skin, soft-tissue, and bone cultures are collected from sites of suspected infection due to trauma, irritation, bites, burns, natural openings, or poor postoperative healing. Wound culture specimens are collected from **superficial wounds** of the epidermis and dermal layers of skin such as rashes, dermatitis lesions, or pustules. The wound surface should be free of debris and disinfected, and then a swab should be used to collect material from the deepest available area of the wound to avoid contamination from normal flora. **Deep-wound** specimens are collected from abscesses, ulcers, and boils in the subcutaneous tissue. The area can be debrided and a specimen collected using the same method noted for superficial wounds. An abscess or boil may also have purulent material expressed and can be collected with a swab or aspirated with a sterile syringe for culture. **Surgical extraction** and **biopsy** may be necessary for collecting deep-tissue samples for culture because they hold the greatest potential to cause a systemic infection. Portions of bone or infected tissue can be debrided, removed, and placed in a sterile cup with a small amount of sterile fluid. Samples suspected of infections caused by anaerobic organisms should be transported in media that reduce O_2 exposure and support the viability of such organisms.

INDIGENOUS ORGANISMS AND MAJOR PATHOGENS OF SKIN, SOFT TISSUE, AND BONE

Soft tissues of the body comprise various structures including muscles, tendons, ligaments, fascia, nerves, fibrous tissues, fat, blood vessels, and synovial membranes. These soft tissues, located deep in the body, and bones are normally sterile. Indigenous skin flora, their Gram stain, and colony morphology on sheep blood agar are described below:

- Gram-positive cocci:
  - *S. aureus*: soft, opaque or pale gold, and circular
  - *S. epidermidis*: opaque, gray, smooth, raised, nonhemolytic
- Gram-positive bacilli in a "Chinese letter" formation:
  - *Propionibacterium acnes*: pigmented white or red, semiopaque, convex, and glistening

Major pathogens and their colony morphologies are described below:

- Aerobic organisms on sheep blood agar:
  - *E. coli*: circular, dull gray, smooth, convex
  - *Klebsiella* species: grayish-white, translucent to opaque, mucoid, circular, dome shaped
  - *P. mirabilis*: pale white, with swarming growth in waves forming concentric circles
  - *P. aeruginosa*: grayish-white, translucent to opaque, circular with irregular edges
  - *S. pyogenes* (group A strep): grayish-white, transparent to translucent, matte or glossy, large zone of hemolysis
  - *S. agalactiae* (group B strep): larger than group A colonies, translucent to opaque, flat, glossy, narrow zone of beta-hemolysis; some strains are nonhemolytic
  - *S. aureus*: soft, opaque or pale gold, and circular
  - *Salmonella* species*: opaque or translucent, smooth, 2–4 mm in diameter
- Facultative anaerobic organisms:
  - *B. fragilis*: gray or white, smooth, shiny, circular on sheep blood agar
  - *Prevotella* species: gray, shiny, circular, turning brown to black after a week of growth on laked blood agar with kanamycin and vancomycin

*Causes osteomyelitis in sickle cell patients. Not a common pathogen in other hosts.

Major Skin, Soft-Tissue, and Bone Infection Pathogens

Many major pathogens of the skin, soft tissues, and bone are also considered parts of the skin's normal flora. However, other pyogenic, or pus-producing, organisms can also cause infections of these tissues. A cut or break in the skin allows bacteria to enter into deeper layers of the skin causing opportunistic infections. Pyogenic organisms release toxic leucocidins that kill host neutrophils and produce pus as a result of accumulating cells and bacteria. *S. aureus* is the most common pathogen causing skin and tissue infections. Infections of the skin and soft tissue are listed below, defined by their site of and cause of infection:

- **Impetigo:** infection affecting healthy superficial skin
- **Cellulitis:** infection of the deeper layers of the skin and soft tissues, occurs on any part of the body
- **Erysipelas:** *S. pyogenes* infection of superficial cutaneous skin on the face or legs only
- **Folliculitis:** localized infection of one hair follicle
- **Boil, furuncle:** painful, hardened, and red bump associated with deep hair follicle infection
- **Carbuncle:** red, swollen, and painful cluster of furuncles under the skin
- **Abscess:** acute or chronic inflammation with a localized collection of pus
- **Osteomyelitis** is a bacterial infection of the bone tissue. Bacteria reach the bone through the bloodstream, introduction of skin flora by recent surgery or open fracture, intravenous drug use, or as an extension of a local injury from the following sources: soft tissues, urogenital tract, or upper and lower respiratory tract.

Genital Tract

Genital Cultures

Commercial collection kits contain the supplies required for specimen collection and transport including a sterile swab with a plastic shaft and a Dacron or rayon tip and a sterile transport tube with the appropriate media to sustain organism viability. Stuart media and Amies charcoal media are often used for the preservation of organisms detected in genital tract samples. Genital tract specimens are collected with the following methods:

- **Urethral** collection is best when preformed more than 1 hour after urination. After discharge is removed from the opening of the urethra, a sterile swab is inserted 2–4 cm into the urethra, rotated for 2–3 seconds to ensure adequate sampling, and then the swab is removed.
- **Vaginal** collection requires excess discharge to be wiped from the opening of the vaginal canal before a swab is inserted. Once inserted into the vaginal canal, the swab is rotated to collect secretions from the mucosal membranes.
- **Cervical** and **endocervical** collection uses a speculum to view the cervical canal; however, lubrication cannot be used when inserting the device because it can be harmful to organisms for culture. Mucus and vaginal material are removed with a swab that is then discarded. A second sterile swab is inserted into the cervix, and the canal is swabbed in a firm but gentle manner. Endocervical samples for chlamydia require more vigorous swabbing to collect epithelial cells.

Indigenous Organisms of Genital Tract

In healthy individuals, most of the internal organs of the genitourinary tract, the kidneys, bladder, ureters, testes, and ovaries, are sterile environments. However, the lower portion of the male and female urethra are inhabited by common normal skin flora, and the female vagina has indigenous species of its own. The following are organisms that comprise the urogenital tract normal flora, along with their corresponding Gram stain and colony morphologies on sheep blood agar:

- Male and female urethra:
  - Gram-positive cocci
    - ❖ *S. epidermidis*: opaque, gray, smooth, raised, nonhemolytic
    - ❖ *Enterococcus faecalis*: small, smooth, gray nonhemolytic
  - Gram-positive bacilli
    - ❖ *Corynebacterium* species: small to medium, gray, white, or yellow, nonhemolytic
  - Gram-negative diplococci
    - ❖ *Neisseria* species: small, white to gray-brown, smooth, butter-like, translucent with a green hue on agar underneath
- Vagina:
  - Gram-positive cocci
    - ❖ *Staphylococcus* species: opaque, white to yellow, smooth, circular
    - ❖ *Micrococcus* species: opaque, white to bright yellow, smooth, raised
    - ❖ *Viridans streptococci*: gray, translucent, umbonate center, alpha-hemolytic
    - ❖ *Enterococcus* species: small, gray, circular
  - Gram-positive bacilli
    - ❖ *Lactobacillus* species: small to medium, gray, alpha-hemolytic
    - ❖ *Corynebacterium* species: see description above
  - Gram-negative bacilli
    - ❖ *Escherichia coli*: circular, dull gray, smooth, convex.

METHODS FOR DETECTION OF PATHOGENS ASSOCIATED WITH VAGINITIS
DETECTION OF TRICHOMONAS

Trichomonas vaginalis can be detected in fresh-void urine from males and females, prostatic secretions, and the vaginal canal. The most common detection of *Trichomonas* is through direct observation on a **wet mount** or in urine sediment. A small amount of sample and a drop of saline are added to a glass slide, and a coverslip is placed on the slide. Microscopic detection of *Trichomonas* reveals a pear-shaped trophozoite similar in size to a neutrophil, moving by its flagella in jerky, undulating movements. If microscopic analysis cannot immediately be observed, *Trichomonas* is still detectable, but it may not be motile and will take on a more spherical shape making it more difficult to differentiate from a WBC. **Immunochromatographic dipsticks** that detect *T. vaginalis* antigens are available, and they eliminate the need for live organisms and immediate testing.

DETECTION OF CANDIDA

Candida species can be detected under microscopic examination using a variety of methods and stains. Yeast can be observed directly with a light microscope in wet mount or urine sediment samples. The use of **KOH** reagent will lyse cells and clear excess debris from samples, aiding in the visualization of yeast and fungal elements. **Calcofluor-white** stain is used to detect yeast species under a UV microscope by fluorescing fungal elements as a bright-white color that is easily visualized. Easily distinguishable from bacteria, *Candida* presents on a Gram stain as Gram-positive buds, pseudohyphae, or true hyphae. A culture and biochemical testing of urine and vaginal samples containing *Candida* organisms can be used to determine the specific species of yeast responsible for the infection.

DETECTION OF BACTERIAL VAGINOSIS

Bacterial vaginosis (BV) is most commonly associated with an overgrowth of *Gardnerella vaginalis*, but it can be caused by up to 35 unique species of aerobic and anaerobic bacteria. The presence of **clue cells** in urine sediment or on a wet mount are indicative of a BV infection. Clue cells are vaginal squamous epithelial cells that are covered in bacteria, giving the cytoplasm a lacy appearance. Wet-prep samples will exhibit clusters of sloughed-off clue cells covered in Gram-variable bacilli and coccobacilli. A Gram stain of a vaginal swab positive for BV will show mixed flora with a decrease in the normal vaginal flora, *Lactobacillus* species. Although more advanced methods are available, the mix of flora shown on a Gram stain can be enumerated and a diagnosis of BV may be made. Molecular PCR methods are also available for detecting species of bacteria known to cause BV.

CULTURE DETECTION

DETECTION OF NEISSERIA GONORRHOEAE AND CHLAMYDIA TRACHOMATIS

N. gonorrhoeae is a fastidious organism with specific storage and growth requirements for culture. Specimens collected for *N. gonorrhoeae* culture should be set up as soon as possible for the best viability of the organism. If inoculating the medium is delayed, samples suspected for a gonorrheal infection must stay at room temperature because refrigeration destroys viable organism. This organism may take up to 48 hours to grow, requires the enrichment of chocolate and Thayer–Martin agars, and must be incubated in a 5–10% CO_2 environment.

C. trachomatis is an incredibly fastidious organism that requires complex and extensive nutrients for cultivation and growth. Due to its intracellular obligations, *C. trachomatis* requires a host cell, such as McCoy cells, to properly grow in a culture setting. Cells are inoculated with sample, incubated in 5–10% CO_2 for 48–72 hours, and observed for brown intracellular growth. Samples suspected of chlamydial infections should be submitted to the lab immediately or frozen at –70 °C for organisms to remain viable.

DETECTION OF STREPTOCOCCUS AGALACTIAE

Women in the third trimester of pregnancy are screened for *Streptococcus agalactiae*, or group B strep, colonization in their vaginal canal and rectum. Infants are able to contract a group B strep infection during delivery that can cause sepsis if not treated promptly and properly. Samples for culture of group B strep are inoculated onto sheep blood agar with vertical stabs made in the agar to promote hemolysis, and they are incubated overnight in 5–10% CO_2. *S. agalactiae* is indicated by colony growth with a narrow zone of beta-hemolysis underneath each colony. A CAMP test can be performed on sheep blood agar to distinguish group B strep from other beta-hemolytic streptococcus species. Diffusible extracellular CAMP proteins produced by *S. agalactiae* react with beta-lysin produced by *S. aureus* to create an arrowhead-shaped zone of hemolysis at the intersection of an *S. agalactiae* streak made perpendicular to a streak of *S. aureus*.

MOLECULAR DETECTION OF *N. GONORRHOEAE*, *C. TRACHOMATIS*, AND *S. AGALACTIAE*

Molecular methods for the detection of *N. gonorrhoeae*, *C. trachomatis*, and *S. agalactiae* are advantageous because they do not rely on organisms' viability and are more specific and time efficient than culture methods. Probe technologies use hybridization and amplification of the bacterial genetic material to detect its presence in samples. **Hybridization** detects bacterial ribosomal RNA with the use of chemiluminescent DNA probes or an RNA/DNA hybrid using antibody-mediated recognition. Some hybridization techniques allow for the detection of *N. gonorrhoeae* and *C. trachomatis* to be determined from a single sample. **Amplification** methods are more sensitive by employing the detection and amplification of nucleic acids in organism-specific genes. **PCR** methods are able to detect small amounts of DNA or RNA in a sample and replicate, or amplify, a target nucleic acid sequence for the detection of specific organisms.

COMMON GENITOURINARY TRACT PATHOGENS

Infections of the genitourinary tract are commonly caused by opportunistic pathogens and manifest into urethritis, vaginitis, and cervicitis. Bacterial vaginitis is a polymicrobial infection that occurs when the balance of normal vaginal flora is disrupted. Vaginitis can also develop from the sexual transmission of the parasite *Trichomonas vaginalis*. Opportunistic fungal infections caused by *Candida albicans* arise when normal flora are inhibited by the use of antibiotics, and these infections often lead to itching, irritation, thick discharge, and burning while urinating. Sexual transmission of *N. gonorrhoeae* and *C. trachomatis* will also lead to genitourinary tract infections and are causative agents in pelvic inflammatory disease that may induce infertility in women. Other common symptoms of gonorrheal and chlamydial infections include lower abdominal pain, discharge from the penis in males, vaginal discharge in females, and painful urination. Herpes simplex virus type 1 (HSV-1) and herpes simplex virus type 2 (HSV-2) are spread by sexual contact causing itching, bumps, rashes, or sores near the genitals, as well as painful urination. Syphilis infections caused by the sexual transmission of *Treponema pallidum* begin with enlarged lymph nodes near the groin and painless sores on the body and genitals. If not treated, syphilis infections can progress into its secondary, latent, and tertiary stages that lead to irreversible systemic damage.

CULTURE AND MOLECULAR DETECTION OF MYCOPLASMA SPECIES

Urine, urethral, vaginal, and endocervical swabs are appropriate samples for detecting *Mycoplasma* species that are responsible for infections of the genital tract. Both culture and molecular methods are available for detection of these organisms. Culture of *Mycoplasma* organisms requires sterol-enriched media containing cholesterol and fatty acids from human or horse serum and incubation at 35–37 °C in a 95% nitrogen and 5% carbon dioxide environment. This slow-growing organism may take up to four weeks after culture setup to grow small colonies with an inverted, "fried egg" appearance. Although culture methods are highly specific for *Mycoplasma* species, they are time-consuming and require expertly trained staff for their cultivation.

Molecular detection of *Mycoplasma* has become the method of choice for testing due to its high sensitivity and increased time efficiency. Real-time PCR and nucleic acid amplification methods have been established for the rapid diagnosis of *Mycoplasma* infections in the genital tract. These methods target and amplify a specific gene or nucleic acid sequence of *Mycoplasma* for the detection of specific organisms. *Mycoplasma genitalium*, a common cause of genital tract infections, is detected molecularly via the *tuf* gene.

VIRULENCE MECHANISMS

Infections of the genital tract are caused by the following organisms whose pathogenicity and virulence factors are described below:

Chlamydia trachomatis functions in two forms: an infectious, extracellular elementary body and a noninfectious, intracellular reticulate body. The elementary body is responsible for adhering to and entering host cells, whereas the reticulate body is the metabolically active form responsible for the intracellular reproduction of bacteria. Major outer membrane protein enzymes allow elementary bodies to evade host defenses extracellularly, whereas the infection thrives intracellularly due to chlamydial proteasome degrading host cell DNA.

Gardnerella vaginalis adheres to host epithelial cells and becomes cytotoxic to these cells with vaginolysin. Sialidase is critical to the organism's survival because it aids in colonization and the formation of a bacterial biofilm within a host.

Neisseria gonorrhoeae possesses pili that aid in organism adherence to host mucosal cells and express antiphagocytic properties. Host IgA antibodies normally block bacterial adhesion; however, IgA protease enzymes in the bacteria hydrolyze IgA, allowing adhesion of host cells to occur and an infection to establish.

Treponema pallidum's adherence to host cells is promoted by outer membrane proteins and infiltration into host cells is facilitated by hyaluronidase. Fibronectin prevents the organism from phagocytosis by macrophages.

URINE

URINE SAMPLES

Random samples may be collected at any time, with no additional preparation or cleansing. Samples of this nature may be used for urine chemistry testing (creatinine, total protein, electrolytes, microalbumin), but they are to be avoided for routine urinalysis or culture testing due to the possibility of erroneous results and an increased chance of contamination.

Midstream clean catch collection comprises cleansing the skin near and around the urethra. Following cleansing, the patient will void first into the toilet and then collect the remaining urine (or an adequate amount) into a collection cup. This method is ideal for urinalysis, bacterial culture, and sensitivity testing.

Catheterized specimens are collected by passing a hollow tube, or catheter, through the urethra and into the bladder. This technique is most commonly used for bacterial culture testing, but it may be used for other routine tests as well.

Suprapubic samples are collected in a sterile environment when a needle is placed through the abdomen and into the bladder. Aspirated urine provides a sterile sample that is free of outside contamination and is ideal for bacterial cultures and cytologic examination.

Nephrostomy tubes are catheters placed through the skin and directly into the kidney. They are used to drain or collect urine when output through the ureters in not possible. Samples may be used for routine urinalysis testing or bacterial culture.

COLONY COUNTS IN URINE CULTURES

Colony counts are extremely important to the process of evaluating urine cultures. Following inoculation and incubation, media are observed for the growth of bacterial colonies, colonies are enumerated, and they are reported as follows:

Observation	Report*
No colony growth	<1,000 colonies
<10	1,000
10	10,000
100	100,000
>100	>100,000

*The colony count is in colony forming units per mL = (number of colonies) × 100.

No growth observed on media after 48 hours of incubation is expected in normal clean-catch, catheterized, suprapubic aspirate and in surgically obtained urine samples. **Fewer than 10 colonies** observed is not considered a significant finding in clean-catch or catheterized specimens, and no further workup is needed. However, any bacterial growth of urine collected from sterile sources is significant and requires further investigation. Cultures with **colony counts between 10 and 100** may be tested further if a patient is having symptoms indicative of a urinary tract infection (UTI). Correlation with other laboratory findings and the patient's clinical signs will influence the decision to test further or not. Growth of **>100 colonies of mixed organisms** exhibiting one predominant organism is a significant finding, and the predominant bacteria will be tested further. Cultures containing three or more organisms with no predominant one indicates a contaminated specimen, no further testing is done, and the collection of a new sample is suggested. A colony count **>100 of a pure, single organism** is indicative of a UTI, and further workup is required to properly identify the organism and perform antibiotic sensitivity testing for guide treatment options.

CORRELATION BETWEEN URINALYSIS RESULTS AND URINE CULTURE EVALUATION

Microscopic and macroscopic urinalysis findings are evaluated and correlated with urine culture findings in the determination of UTIs. Nitrite, pH, and leukocyte esterase chemical reactions on a urine dipstick indicate the presence or absence of bacteria in a sample. Common UTI-causing bacteria, including *E. coli*, *Klebsiella*, *Proteus*, *Pseudomonas*, and *Enterobacter* species, will reduce nitrate to nitrite, creating a **positive nitrite** dipstick result. Leukocyte esterase is an enzyme found in neutrophils, and a **positive leukocyte esterase** result indicates a UTI because WBCs are commonly found in areas of infection. An **alkaline pH** may indicate the presence of infection-causing bacteria in urine because some bacteria hydrolyze urea into the alkaline substance ammonia. Macroscopic observations of **WBCs** and **bacteria** in urine sediment are also correlated with urine culture results in the determination of a UTI. The noted urinalysis results alone are only indications of an infection and provide guidance in culture evaluation. Following urinalysis results, urine culture growth, quantification, and organism identification are used to confirm or deny the presence of a UTI.

IDENTIFICATION METHODS (THEORY, INTERPRETATION, AND APPLICATION)
COLONY MORPHOLOGY ON MICROBIOLOGY CULTURES

A bacterial colony is a visible mass of identical organisms that grows from a single bacterial cell. Different genera, species, and strains of bacteria present with distinct visual appearances that are used as the first step in isolating and identifying infectious agents. Evaluating colony morphology also aids in determining the purity of a culture by more easily recognizing contamination of other organisms. Within 18–24 hours after being inoculated with sample, organisms growing on microbiology media are visually observed. A hand lens or magnifying glass can be used to aid in identifying key characteristics. Colony morphology is evaluated by the following characteristics:

- Colony size
- Form and margins
- Elevation
- Surface features, texture, and consistency
- Color, transparency, and iridescence.

CATEGORIZATION AND INTERPRETATION OF COLONY MORPHOLOGY CHARACTERISTICS

Colony morphology is categorized by size, form, margins, and elevation characteristics in the following ways:

- **Colony size** is categorized by diameter:
  - Pinpoint or punctiform < 1 mm
  - Small 1–2 mm
  - Medium 3–4 mm
  - Large > 5 mm

The form, margins, and elevation of a colony give it a distinctive shape:

- **Forms** are categorized as
  - Circular, symmetrical circle
  - Irregular, lacking symmetry
  - Filamentous, exhibiting threadlike branching
  - Rhizoid, exhibiting a branching, rootlike shape
- The **margins**, or edges, of a colony are most commonly evaluated as

  - Entire, meaning smooth
  - Undulate, meaning wavy
  - Lobular, fingerlike growth spreading outward
  - Scalloped, rounded projections resembling a scallop shell
  - Filiform, thin and wavy layers spreading outward.
- The **elevation** of bacterial colonies refers to its cross-sectional shape. Colony elevations are categorized by the following shapes:
  - Flat
  - Raised
  - Convex, curved or rounded upward
  - Crateriform, sunken in the middle
  - Umbonate, with the middle protruding upward.

Surface texture and consistency are described as having the following characteristics:

- **Textures** are described with the following terms:
  - Smooth,
  - Wrinkled, shriveled
  - Rough, granular
  - Dull, no shine
  - Glistening, shining
- The **consistency** of colonies is described as the following:
  - Moist
  - Dry
  - Viscid, thick and sticky
  - Mucoid, moist and sticky
  - Butyrous, butter-like

Colonies can exhibit a variety of transparencies and pigmentations:

- Colony **transparency** is categorized as
  - Transparent, clear, see-through
  - Translucent, semiclear, frosted-glass appearance
  - Opaque, unable to see through
  - Iridescent, color changing in reflective light
- Sheep blood and chocolate agars often yield the following **colony colors**:
  - White
  - Cream
  - Yellow
- Differential and selective medias can produce many colors based on the organism's biochemical properties such as:
  - Pink
  - Green
  - Blue
  - Black

RAPID TESTS USED FOR PRESUMPTIVE IDENTIFICATION
CATALASE AND COAGULASE TESTS

The following rapid tests are used for presumptive identification of organisms:

- **Catalase:** This test is used to determine the presence of the catalase enzyme in an organism and differentiate catalase-positive staphylococci from catalase-negative streptococci organisms. An organism colony is placed on a glass slide, followed by a drop of 3% hydrogen peroxide. If catalase is present, the enzyme will break down hydrogen peroxide into O_2 and water.
  - **Catalase positive**: bubbling produced
  - **Catalase negative**: no visible bubbling
- **Coagulase:** This test is used to differentiate coagulase-positive *S. aureus* from other *Staphylococcus* species. Commercial kits are available to detect bound coagulase, or clumping factor, by adding reagent rabbit plasma to an organism colony on a glass slide. If present, bound coagulase and protein A on the cell wall agglutinates with reagent for a positive reaction.
  - **Coagulase positive**: visible clumping on the slide.
  - **Coagulase negative**: no visible clumping or agglutination. Free or unbound coagulase can be detected in a tube with gel containing rabbit plasma. The presence of free coagulase will form a visible fibrin clot after 4 hours of incubation at 35 °C. If no clot is observed at 4 hours, incubation is extended to 24 hours.

OXIDASE AND INDOLE TESTS

The following rapid tests are used for the presumptive identification of organisms:

- **Oxidase:** This test is used for a presumptive identification of *Neisseria* species and *P. aeruginosa*. A colony of organism is added to filter paper impregnated with Kovac's oxidase reagent (tetramethyl-*p*-phenylenediamine), and a color change, or lack of, is observed. Organisms producing the cytochrome oxidase enzyme will oxidize the reagent indicating a positive test result, whereas organisms that do not produce the enzyme will be oxidase negative.
  - **Oxidase positive:** development of a dark-purple color within 10 seconds
  - **Oxidase negative:** colorless, or remains the original color of the colony
- **Indole:** This test is used for a presumptive identification of *E. coli* and differentiation of swarming *Proteus* species. Organisms that produce the enzyme tryptophanase break down tryptophan amino acids, yielding indole. Filter paper is saturated with indole reagent, and a colony of organism is rubbed onto the filter paper. Indole-positive organisms are determined by indole's ability to combine with indicator aldehydes to form a color compound.
  - **Indole positive**: rapid development of a blue or green-blue color
  - **Indole negative**: no color change.

PYR AND UREASE TESTS

The following rapid tests are used for presumptive identification of organisms:

- **PYR**: This test is used to identify *Enterococcus* species and group A beta-hemolytic streptococci through the presence of the enzyme pyrrolidonyl. Filter paper is impregnated with the substrate PYR that is acted on by pyrrolidonyl. The paper is inoculated with the organism being tested, the color developing reagent N,N-dimethylaminocinnamaldehyde is added, and the results are interpreted after 5 minutes.
  - **PYR positive:** development of a bright-red color
  - **PYR negative:** no color change, or a yellow-orange color
- **Urease:** This test is used to detect *C. neoformans* in sputum samples and differentiate pathogenic *Shigella* and *Salmonella* species from nonpathogenic *Proteus* species in stool cultures. Urease-producing organisms hydrolyze urea-releasing ammonia that changes the alkalinity of a sample placed on pH paper. The production of ammonia reacts with the phenol red indicator and causes a color change in urease-positive organisms.
  - **Urease positive:** color change to magenta
  - **Urease negative:** no color change, pH paper remains yellow.

CONVENTIONAL BIOCHEMICAL IDENTIFICATION

TRIPLE SUGAR IRON (TSI) AGAR

A triple sugar iron (**TSI**) agar slant is used for presumptive identification of many Gram-negative bacilli, most commonly the enteric pathogens in the *Enterobacteriaceae* family. This method is based on an organism's ability or inability to produce gas and H_2S and to ferment certain sugars. TSI agar contains the following:

- Sugars — glucose, lactose, and sucrose
- Nutrient source — peptone
- Sulfur source — sodium thiosulfate

51

- Indicator — ferric ammonium citrate
- pH indicator — phenol red.

TSI is inoculated using a needle carrying a pure colony of the organism to be identified. The needle is stabbed through the middle of the agar and into the bottom, or **butt**, of the agar. The **slant** is also inoculated by streaking the organism along its surface while removing the needle. TSI is interpreted after 18–24 hours of incubation at 35 °C.

The following characteristics and changes observed in TSI are as follows:

Notation	Color Change	Metabolic Change
K/K	Slant, red; butt, red	No sugars fermented, no reaction
K/A	Slant, red; butt, yellow	Glucose fermented; lactose and sucrose not fermented
A/A	Slant, yellow; butt, yellow	Glucose fermented; lactose, sucrose, or both fermented
G	Bubbles/splitting in the butt of the agar	Gas production
H_2S	Black precipitate	H_2S production

DECARBOXYLASE TESTING

Decarboxylase testing, also called Moeller's method, measures an organism's ability to hydrolyze an amino acid to form an amine and often aids in the identification of organisms of the *Enterobacteriaceae* family. Hydrolysis of the carboxyl portion of an amino acid to form an alkaline-reacting amine produces a change in color in the test tubes.

For testing, a very heavy suspension is prepared by combining brain heart infusion broth with a young colony of organism that has been grown on 5% sheep blood agar for 18–24 hours. Three decarboxylase broths containing arginine, lysine, and ornithine and a control broth with no amino acid added are then inoculated with the suspension. Glucose-nonfermenting organisms will be inoculated with four drops of organism suspension, and glucose-fermenting organisms will be inoculated with one drop. Cover the medium with a 4 mm layer of sterile mineral oil, incubate at 35–37 °C, and examine at 24, 48, 72, and 96 hours of incubation.

- **Decarboxylase positive**: purple color change compared to orange in the control tube
- **Decarboxylase negative**: No color change, or yellow color in the test and control tubes.

CARBOHYDRATE UTILIZATION TESTING

Carbohydrate utilization testing is performed to definitively identify yeast species in clinical specimens. Yeasts and yeast-like fungi can be identified by a carbohydrate utilization profile because they each use specific carbohydrate substrates. To perform carbohydrate utilization testing, a yeast is combined with saline or distilled water to create a 4.0 McFarland standard suspension. The suspension is then used to cover the surface of a yeast nitrogen base agar plate containing bromocresol purple and is allowed to dry. Sterile forceps are used to place selected carbohydrate disks about 30 mm apart on the surface of the agar. After 24–48 hours of incubation at 30 °C, the plate is observed for carbohydrate utilization by the presence of a color change or growth around a disk. The results obtained by carbohydrate utilization tests create a profile for the organism tested that is compared to profiles established in mycology laboratory manuals for organism identification.

- **Carbohydrate utilization positive**: color change or growth around the disk
- **Carbohydrate utilization negative**: no color change or growth around the disk.

52

MOTILITY TESTING

Motility testing is done to determine if an organism is motile or not, allowing for further differentiation among organisms. There are two methods for determining motility, the hanging drop method and the semisolid agar method. Each method's procedure and interpretation are as follows:

Hanging drop:

- Use a 25 °C, actively growing, 6- to 24-hour-old broth culture.
- Place one drop of culture into the center of a coverslip.
- Place one drop of immersion oil on each corner of the coverslip.
- Place a depression slide on top of the coverslip, allowing the corners to seal, and invert the slide with the coverslip on top and the sample in the convex portion of the slide.
- Examine with the 40× objective.
- Interpretation:
  - **Positive:** true motility — organisms change position in respect to one another, commonly darting across the field.
  - **Negative:** organisms appear active, but they remain in the same position relative to other organisms and debris.

Semisolid agar:

- Using a straight needle, touch an 18- to 24-hour old colony growing on agar medium.
- Stab a needle 1/3 to 1/2 of the depth of the agar in the middle of the tube.
- Incubate 35–37 °C, and examine daily for up to 7 days.
- Interpretation:
  - **Positive:** from the site of inoculation, organisms will spread out into the medium.
  - **Negative:** organisms will remain at the site of inoculation.

X AND V FACTORS

X and V factor testing is done to aid in the identification and differentiation of *Haemophilus* species based on the organisms' use of the growth factors. X factor consists of hemin, whereas V factor is composed of NAD. *H. influenzae* is the most important organism identified by this test because it can cause meningitis and pneumonia.

This test begins with a light suspension of organism in saline. A sterile swab is dipped into the suspension and rolled across the surface of a trypticase soy agar plate. X, V, and XV factor disks are placed 4–5 cm apart on the agar's surface. The agar is incubated at 35 °C, and organism growth is observed and evaluated the next day:

- **Positive**:
  - X and V: growth around the XV disk only
  - V factor: growth around the V disk, light growth around the XV disk, and no growth around the X disk
  - X factor: growth around the X disk, light growth around the XV disk, and no growth around the V disk
- **Negative:** growth over the entire surface of the agar

COMMERCIAL KITS USED IN MICROBIOLOGY TESTING

Commercial test kits are used for the rapid detection of various microbiologic pathogens. The following methodologies are commonly used:

- **Latex agglutination** kits allow for qualitative and semiquantitative evaluation of virulent organisms such as meningitis-causing *Cryptococcus*. Reagent latex beads are coated in organism-specific antibodies and are then combined with the patient sample. Agglutination between reagent antibodies and organism surface antigens represents the presence of the organism in question.
- **Monoclonal antibody** test kits are also used in microbiology testing for antigens produced by *H. pylori* or toxins given off by toxigenic *C. difficile*. If the target organism or toxin is present in a sample, it will attach to reagent antibodies imbedded in the test cartridge. The antigen–antibody complex formed will migrate to the test window and produce a colored line.

AUTOMATED TESTING METHODS USED IN MICROBIOLOGY LABS

Automated systems are used in microbiology for blood culture monitoring, organism identification, and antibiotic susceptibility testing. Incubated systems continuously monitor blood culture bottles for chemical reactions that indicate bacterial growth. Carbon dioxide (CO_2) generation is indicative of bacterial growth in blood culture bottles, and automated systems will alert of a positive blood culture when a specific CO_2 threshold is passed. Organism identification and antibiotic susceptibility testing are achieved with instrumentation comprised of the following components: incubator, automated reader, data terminal, printer, and the ability to be connected to the LIS. Panels used for these systems are plastic trays with microwells coated in biochemical or antibiotic-specific reagents that are inoculated with a suspension of bacteria. Panels are available based on organism Gram stains and growth requirements to optimize the identification of an isolate. Turbidity, colorimetry, and fluorescent or matrix-assisted laser desorption ionization time-of-flight mass spectrometry (MALDI-TOF MS) methods are used to determine biochemical reactions that are compared to those of known isolates in the instrument's computerized database. Automated systems allow for rapid and confident identification of pathogens.

Automated specimen processing and total automation systems have been developed for the microbiology laboratory, with conveyors, streaking mechanisms, and incubators, among other technologies. However, automated systems rely on classic time-consuming culture techniques and require extensive knowledge for handling the various types of microbiological specimens.

MATRIX-ASSISTED LASER DESORPTION IONIZATION TIME-OF-FLIGHT MASS SPECTROMETRY

Matrix-assisted laser desorption ionization time-of-flight mass spectrometry (MALDI-TOF MS) provides microbial identification and characterization in a fast, precise, and cost-effective manner. MALDI-TOF MS allows for organism identification even in a mixed colony culture, but it does not provide antibiotic susceptibility information.

This method is divided into two phases: ionization and time of flight. Ionization consists of a sample being fixed to a crystalline matrix and bombarded by a laser. The laser vaporizes molecules into a vacuum and ionizes without decomposing or fragmenting them. The TOF MS phase of the process separates ions based on their mass-to-charge ratio and determines the time that each molecule takes to reach a detector. Molecular patterns are profiled and compared to profiles of known microbes to identify and characterize an organism.

MULTIPLEX MOLECULAR METHODS

Multiplex molecular methods allow for testing of multiple pathogens at the same time aiding in detecting infections that may otherwise go undiagnosed. PCR molecular methodology is used with the presence of multiple primer pairs specific to various bacteria, viruses, and parasites. A primer for each pathogen in a multiplex system is 18–22 base pairs in size, establishes specificity for the pathogen, and requires primers of similar melting points for the best results. The detection and amplification of multiple targets in one test cycle are advantageous for microbiology testing by requiring a smaller sample and less time to diagnose a patient and begin appropriate care. Most commonly, multiplex systems are used in the detection of respiratory or gastrointestinal pathogens that are highly contagious and are difficult to differentiate from one another based on their clinical signs and symptoms.

GENETIC SEQUENCING

Genetic sequencing methodologies target variable regions on the 16s ribosomal RNA gene in individual bacteria for classification and identification purposes. Many bacterial genus and species react and present similarly using traditional culture and identification methods, making it difficult to distinguish one from the other and to determine a specific cause for a disease. Genetic sequencing uses primer tools to amplify the following variable regions on the 16s gene on the bacterial genome: V2, V3, V4, V6, V7, V8, and V9. Amplification of these regions allows for the identification of bacterial organisms down to the genus and species level. Genetic sequences for bacterial are collected and stored in a database that provides laboratories with a reference for bacterial identification. Gene sequencing does not require single isolates or bacterial colonies grown in culture. Bacterial genomes can be sequenced directly from the samples collected and can be performed on mixed microbial samples.

ANTIMICROBIAL SUSCEPTIBILITY TESTING AND ANTIBIOTIC RESISTANCE
ANTIMICROBIAL SUSCEPTIBILITY AND RESISTANCE TESTING

Antimicrobial susceptibility and antibiotic resistance testing is required to find the correct agent and the appropriate concentration to eliminate a bacterial infection. The most commonly used testing methods are dilutions and disk diffusion, but automated methods are also widely available and used. If automated methods are unclear or raise questions, traditional diffusion and dilution methods are used to clarify any discrepancies. **Broth dilution** methods require multiple tubes containing varying concentrations of antibiotics with a suspension of the test isolate added. Organism growth in each dilution is observed for the determination of minimum inhibitory concentration (MIC) and minimum bactericidal concentration. The **MIC** is the lowest concentration of drug necessary to inhibit organism growth and multiplication. The lowest concentration of a drug that will result in the death of a bacterial population is known as the **minimum bactericidal concentration. Disk diffusion** methods determine antibiotic resistance or susceptibility by observing the zone of bacterial growth inhibition surrounding antibiotic-impregnated disks on culture media. A result of no bacterial growth, or **susceptible**, indicates that the organism will most likely will respond to treatment with the agent. **Intermediate** growth indicates that a high dose of agent may be necessary for successful treatment, whereas no zone of inhibition indicates antibiotic **resistance** and that treatment with an agent will most likely fail. Antimicrobial susceptibility and antibiotic resistance testing is an important step in the process of treating patient infections, and the tests in vivo are an estimate of the effectiveness that the agent will have against an organism in vivo.

PHENOTYPIC DETECTION OF RESISTANCE

BETA-LACTAMASE

The **beta-lactamase**, or **nitrocefin, test** is a rapid method that detects the presence of beta-lactamase enzyme production in strains of *S. aureus, N. gonorrhoeae, Moraxella. catarrhalis,* and *H. influenzae.* Beta-lactamase enzymes hydrolyze the beta-lactam rings of penicillin and cephalosporin antibiotics, rendering them inactive. This method uses paper disks impregnated with nitrocefin, a chromogenic cephalosporin that changes color when the amide bond in the beta-lactam ring is hydrolyzed by the enzyme. The procedure and interpretation of beta-lactamase phenotype testing are described below:

- Procedure
  - Using sterile forceps, place a nitrocefin disk on an empty petri dish or microscope slide.
  - Allow the disk to come to room temperature.
  - Moisten the disk with one drop of sterile deionized water.
  - Use a sterilized loop of applicator stick to remove an isolated colony and spread it on the surface of the disk.
  - Observe the disk for the development of color.
- Interpretation
  - **Positive**, penicillin and cephalosporin resistance: red-orange color
  - **Negative**, penicillin and cephalosporin susceptible: yellow color.

EXTENDED-SPECTRUM BETA-LACTAMASES (ESBLS)

Extended spectrum beta-lactamase (ESBL)-producing strains of *Escherichia* and *Klebsiella* organisms are detected by the **double-disk synergy method**. Organisms possessing the ESBL enzyme are able to hydrolyze the oxyimino side chain of extended-spectrum cephalosporins, rendering them inactive. Therefore, antibiotic options for the treatment of infections caused by these organisms are extremely limited, with carbapenems being the antimicrobial of choice. The procedure and interpretation of double-disk synergy testing for ESBL detection are described below:

- Procedure:
  - Prepare a 0.5 McFarland standard suspension with an ESBL-suspected isolate.
  - Inoculate the entire surface of a Mueller–Hinton agar plate with the suspension.
  - Place a disk impregnated with the third-generation cephalosporin cefotaxime in the middle of the plate.
  - Place an amoxicillin/clavulanate-impregnated disk on the agar roughly 20 mm from the cefotaxime disk.
  - Incubate for 16–18 hours at 37 °C.
- Interpretation:
  - **Positive, extended-spectrum cephalosporin-resistant**: zone of inhibition around the ceftazidime disk expanded by and in the direction of the clavulanate disk
  - **Negative, extended-spectrum cephalosporin-susceptible**: no expanded zone of inhibition

INDUCIBLE CLINDAMYCIN RESISTANCE

The **inducible clindamycin resistance test**, or **D test**, is used to detect inducible clindamycin resistance in strains of *S. aureus* that were clindamycin sensitive and erythromycin resistant. These strains possess enzymes that have the capability to induce resistance during antimicrobial therapy. Routine antibiotic susceptibility testing is unable to detect these strains and may cause a failure in the clinical treatment of MRSA infections. The D test is a disk diffusion method that is able to detect inducible resistance prior to beginning antimicrobial therapy. The D test procedure and interpretation of results are described below:

- Procedure:
  - Prepare a 0.5 McFarland standard suspension with erythromycin-resistant *S. aureus* isolates.
  - Inoculate the entire surface of a Mueller–Hinton agar plate with the suspension.
  - Place a clindamycin disk and an erythromycin disk 15–20 mm apart in the center of the plate.
  - Incubate for 16–18 hours at 37 °C.
- Interpretation:
  - **D phenotype (D+):** a blunt, D-shaped zone of inhibition around the clindamycin disk
  - **Noninduction phenotypes (negative):** a clear, circular zone of inhibition around the clindamycin disk.

CARBAPENAMASES

The **modified Hodge test** detects pathogens possessing the beta-lactamase enzyme, carbapenemase, that inactivates carbapenem and all other beta-lactam antibiotics. Infections caused by carbapenem-resistant *Enterobacteriaceae* (CRE) bacteria are extremely dangerous, and detection is necessary for effective treatment. The principle of this test is based on a carbapenemase-producing test isolate's ability to enable the carbapenem susceptible indictor organism to expand its growth along the test isolate inoculum steak. The modified Hodge test procedure and interpretation of results are described below:

- Procedure:
  - Prepare a 0.5 McFarland standard suspension of the following:
    - ❖ Known, indicator organism, *E. coli*
    - ❖ Suspected CRE test isolate
    - ❖ CRE-positive quality control organism
    - ❖ CRE-negative quality control organism
  - With sterile saline, make a 1:10 dilution of the indicator organism.
  - Inoculate the entire surface of a Mueller–Hinton agar plate with the diluted indicator suspension and allow it to dry for 3–5 minutes.
  - Place a 10 µg meropenem- or ertapenem-impregnated disk in the center of the agar.
  - Streak the test isolate suspension in a straight line from the edge of the disk to the edge of the plate. Repeat this step with each quality-control organism.
  - Incubate for 16–24 hours at 37 °C.
- Interpretation:
  - **Positive, carbapenem resistant:** *E. coli* growth presents with a clover leaf-like indentation at the intersection of the test isolate and *E. coli* in the disk zone of inhibition.
  - **Negative, carbapenem susceptible:** no *E. coli* growth along the test organism streak in the disk diffusion zone.

DETECTION METHODS FOR GENETIC DETERMINANTS OF ANTIMICROBIAL RESISTANCE

Detecting genes with known antibiotic resistant properties is most commonly accomplished with PCR testing, but other molecular methods may be used as well. Genetic determination for drug resistance must be coupled with phenotypic assays to determine the level or extent of resistance present. Below are the test methods used for the genetic detection of drug resistance in pathogenic organisms:

- **mecA** — MRSA
  - **PCR** with gene-specific primers and probes
  - **Enzymatic detection PCR**: enzyme-labeled PCR gene probes are detected by immunosorbent assays
- **vanA** — resistance to high levels of vancomycin
  - **PCR** with gene-specific primers and probes
  - **Pulse-field gel electrophoresis:** separates organism DNA, pattern produced in gel determines the presence or absence of a gene
  - **Multilocus enzyme electrophoresis**: specific proteins are separated in gel, and a probe detects the presence of absence of the proteins
- **blaKPC** — beta-lactamase gene from *K. pneumoniae*
  - **Real-time PCR with fluorescent-labeled probe**: PCR amplification with forward and reverse primers, hybridization of gene DNA, if present, fluorescent probe allows for detection by real-time PCR.

PATTERNS OF INTRINSIC ANTIBIOTIC RESISTANCE EXHIBITED BY COMMON PATHOGENS

Intrinsic resistance to an antibiotic or family of antibiotics occurs naturally in certain organisms without the need for genetic mutation or the acquisition of genes. Naturally occurring mechanisms that induce antibiotic resistance include reduced outer membrane permeability by porins, efflux pumps actively pumping antibiotics out of the bacterial cell, and enzymes inactivating the drug. **Porins** act as pores in the cell wall membrane, allowing molecules in and out of the cell. The size and number of porins present in bacterial cell walls can exclude the entrance of certain sized antibiotic molecules. The structural difference between Gram-positive and Gram-negative organisms' cell walls acts as an intrinsic resistance to penicillin and glycoprotein activity in Gram-negative bacteria because larger molecules cannot pass through the cell wall. Gram-negative bacteria also have **efflux pumps** inside the cell that actively pump out antibiotics that have entered the cell. Through actively removing drugs from the cell, agents are not able to reach the appropriate bactericidal concentration, rendering them ineffective. Gram-negative bacteria use a combination of these mechanisms to cause resistance to different antibiotics.

Examples of common pathogens exhibiting patterns of intrinsic resistance are listed below:

- *E. coli*
  - AcrAB-TolC:
    - ❖ active efflux and inactivation of beta-lactams by beta-lactamase
    - ❖ active efflux and limited uptake of tetracyclines and chloramphenicol
    - ❖ active efflux, modified target, and limited uptake of fluoroquinolones
- *P. aeruginosa*
  - mexAB, mexXY: multidrug-resisting efflux pumps
- *K. pneumoniae*
  - inactivation of beta-lactams by beta-lactamase and plasmids

MECHANISMS OF ACTION OF MAJOR ANTIBIOTIC CLASSES

Antibiotics have been developed for the treatment of various types of microbial infections. Classes of antibiotic act on a unique parts of organisms causing one of two outcomes: **bacteriostatic**, prevention of growth and multiplication of cells, or **bactericidal**, cell death. The major classes of antibiotics, their mechanisms of action, and their expected results on microbes are described as follows:

Beta-lactams bind to the penicillin-binding proteins in the cell wall of Gram-positive and Gram-negative bacteria. Binding to penicillin-binding proteins will inactivate peptidoglycan and cell wall synthesis, causing cell death.

Glycopeptides bind to the peptidoglycan precursor of Gram-positive organisms, inhibiting cell wall synthesis, and causing cell death. This class of antibiotics contains the drugs of choice in severe infections caused by *Clostridium difficile* and methicillin-resistant *S. aureus* (MRSA).

Aminoglycosides bind to bacterial RNA, inhibiting protein synthesis in Gram-negative aerobes and facultative anaerobes and causing cell death.

Tetracyclines and **macrolides** inhibit bacterial protein synthesis of Gram-positive organisms. They function as bacteriostatic agents in patients with moderate infections and those allergic to beta-lactams, by preventing growth and the multiplication of bacterial cells.

Sulfonamides bind to dihydropteroate synthase, which inhibits folate synthesis and prevents the growth and multiplication of various urinary tract and enteric pathogens.

Quinolones inhibit bacterial replication by targeting enzymes required for DNA synthesis, causing cell death. This drug class is often used to treat genitourinary infections and hospital- or community-acquired nosocomial infections.

MRSA/MSSA, VRE, ESBL/CRE SCREENING
SPECIMEN SOURCES

Screening for the colonization of antibiotic-resistant bacteria is common for patients in healthcare facilities. Colonization occurs when the potential pathogen resides in the body with no present signs or symptoms of infection. Patients colonized with these bacteria are at increased risk for severe antibiotic-resistant infections. Resistant bacteria also have the potential to spread from patient to patient in healthcare facilities on the hands of healthcare workers and visitors, body fluids, or contaminated objects and surfaces. Appropriate specimens for the screening of common multidrug-resistant bacteria colonization are described below:

- **Swab of the left and right nares** because staphylococcus bacteria often colonize in the mucous membranes of the nose
  - Methicillin-resistant *S. aureus* **(MRSA)** and methicillin-sensitive *S. aureus* **(MSSA)**
- **Rectal swab** because these bacteria survive and colonize in the gastrointestinal tract
  - Vancomycin-resistant *Enterococci* **(VRE)**
  - Extended-spectrum beta-lactamases **(ESBLs)**
  - Carbapenem-resistant *Enterobacteriaceae* **(CRE)**

CULTURE METHODS

Culture methods available for the screening and detection of antibiotic-resistant organisms use a combination of selective media and antibiotic-impregnated agar or disks. **Chromogenic agar** is a selective media containing nutrients and inhibitors specific to the cultivation of the target organism. If present, target organism colonies can easily be recognized by their color. Culture methods for common antibiotic-resistant organisms are described below:

- MRSA/MSSA
  - **Oxacillin disk on Mueller–Hinton agar**: MRSA exhibits a zone of inhibition ≤10 mm from the disk.
  - Chromogenic agar
- VRE
  - **Bile esculin azide agar with 6µg/mL of vancomycin and confirmatory MIC:** growth of *Enterococci* colonies indicates vancomycin resistance. Colonies appear black on the agar and require MIC testing to confirm resistance.
  - **Brain heart infusion agar with 6 µg/mL of vancomycin:** requires suspension of pure isolate colonies, no bacterial growth after 24 hours of incubation detects vancomycin susceptibility, any bacterial growth confirms resistance.
- ESBL
  - **Third-generation cephalosporin and clavulanic acid disks on Mueller–Hinton agar**: in the presence of clavulanic acid, ESBL organisms will present an increased zone of inhibition on agar.
- CRE
  - Chromogenic agar

MOLECULAR METHODS

Molecular testing is available for the screening and detection of antibiotic resistant organisms colonized in a patient's mucous membranes. Detection of the following bacteria is pertinent to optimizing patient treatment and care: methicillin-resistant *S. aureus* (**MRSA**) versus methicillin-sensitive *S. aureus* (**MSSA**), vancomycin-resistant *Enterococci* (**VRE**), extended-spectrum beta-lactamases (**ESBLs**), and carbapenem-resistant *Enterobacteriaceae* (**CRE**). Antibiotic-resistant organisms are molecularly detected by their expression of specific genes that are responsible for their resistance. MRSA is differentiated from MSSA by the expression of the **mecA gene** that can be detected via PCR methodologies using gene-specific primers and probes or enzyme-labeled gene probes and ELISA techniques. The **vanA gene** expressed by **VRE** organisms can be detected using the following molecular methods: PCR with gene specific primers and probes, pulse-field gel electrophoresis that separates DNA to reveal the presence of absence of vanA, or multilocus enzyme electrophoresis with probes to detect vanA proteins. **Beta-lactamase genes** responsible for **ESBL** organisms' resistance are detected with real-time PCR methodologies using fluorescent labeled probes. Nucleic acid amplification techniques are used to detect one or more **carbapenemase genes** expressed by **CRE** organisms.

ANTIBIOTIC RESISTANT BACTERIA

Antibiotic-resistant bacterial infections can be acquired in the community or in a hospital setting. Hospital-acquired infections are linked to a variety of sources and modes of transmission including the following:

- Surgical or invasive device implantation site
- Central line-associated bloodstream infections
- Catheter-associated UTIs
- Ventilator-associated pneumonia
- Contact with healthcare workers' or visitors' contaminated hands.

These bacteria inhabit parts of the body as normal flora and become pathogens when they are introduced to parts of the body where they don't normally reside. MRSA and MSSA organisms are normally found as commensal organisms on the surface of the skin and mucous membranes, whereas VRE, ESBL, and CRE can colonize in the gastrointestinal tract without causing infection. These bacteria possess all of the virulence factors associated with their antibiotic susceptible strains, as well as genetic mutations and enzymes that resist commonly used antibiotic therapy. Resistance to antibiotics is a growing concern as treating such infections becomes increasingly more difficult.

BIOSAFETY LEVEL 3 PATHOGENS AND SELECT AGENTS (BIOTERRORISM)
SPECIMEN SOURCES OF BIOSAFETY LEVEL 3 PATHOGENS AND AGENTS OF BIOTERRORISM

Biosafety level 3 pathogens are agents that have the potential to cause serious or fatal disease when aerosols are inhaled into the body. Specimens suspected of being biosafety level 3 pathogens require handling under a biological safety cabinet with engineering features to control air movement. Common biosafety level 3 pathogens include tuberculosis and the mold stages of systemic fungi. Specimen sources include sputum and blood.

Specimens suspected of containing agents of bioterrorism must be handled with extreme care and following strict protocols to ensure public safety. Agents of bioterrorism can be recovered in the following clinical specimens:

- Fluid and tissue from cutaneous lesions
- Stool
- Blood
- Sputum

BACILLUS ANTHRACIS

Bacillus anthracis react and present in the following ways:

- **Biochemical reactions:**

Catalase	+
Oxidase	−
Urease	−
TSI	K/K
H_2S	−

Motility	−
Indole	+
Nitrate reduction	+

- **Gram stain:** Gram-positive spore-forming bacilli in a long chain, resembling bamboo shoots
- **Growth requirements:** aerobic, and facultative anaerobe, grow best at 35–37 °C
- **Colony morphology:** nonhemolytic, dry, ground glass surface, with irregular edges, and comma protrusions called "Medusa head" on sheep blood agar
- **Rapid test:** RedLine Alert Test — FDA-approved immunochromatographic kit test for presumptive *B. anthracis* identification from suspicious bacterial colonies grown on sheep blood agar.

YERSINIA PESTIS

Yersinia pestis react and present in the following ways:

- **Biochemical reactions:**

Oxidase	−
Urease	−
Catalase	+
Indole	−
TSI	K/A

- **Gram stain:** Gram-negative bacilli with bipolar staining, resembling a safety pin.
- **Growth requirements:** aerobic and facultative anaerobe, grow best at 25–30 °C.
- **Colony morphology:** pinpoint growth at 24 hours, and rough, cauliflower appearance at 48 hours on sheep blood agar. Colonies are colorless to peach on MacConkey, salmon colored on Hektoen agar, and colorless to yellow on XLD agar.
- **Rapid test:** Presumptive identification of *Y. pestis* can be determined with ELISA or immunochromatographic methodologies that detect a capsular antigen specific to the organism.

BRUCELLA SPECIES

Brucella species react and present in the following ways:

- **Biochemical reactions:**

Oxidase	+
Urease	+
Nitrate	+
Motility	−

- **Gram stain:** Gram-negative coccobacilli, resembling grains of sand.
- **Growth requirements:** aerobic, facultative intracellular parasite, grow best at 37 °C in 5–10% CO_2. Cultures must be incubated for 21–30 days to confirm negative.
- **Colony morphology:** small, smooth, convex, translucent to opaque, nonhemolytic on sheep blood agar. Colonies appear yellow, but they may turn brown as they age.
- **Rapid test:** a particle agglutination test with a positive *Brucella* antibody titer of 1:160 or greater is used as a presumptive identification.

FRANCISELLA TULARENSIS

Francisella tularensis react and present in the following ways:

- **Biochemical reactions:**

Oxidase	−
Urease	−
Catalase	weak +
Beta-lactamase	+
H$_2$S with lead acetate	+

- **Gram stain**: faint staining, Gram-negative pleomorphic coccobacilli
- **Growth requirements**: strict aerobe, requires cysteine for optimal growth at 35–37 °C
- **Colony morphology**: tiny, gray-white on chocolate agar and small, green-blue colonies on cysteine heart agar after 48 hours of growth
- **Rapid test**: fluorescent antibody stains, immunohistological stains, and antibody agglutination tests are available for the identification of *F. tularensis.*

VIRULENCE MECHANISMS

Agents of bioterrorism are incredibly infectious organisms that possess the potential to cause harm to many people in a short amount of time. Due to their ability to transmit via the inhalation of aerosols, Biosafety level 3 pathogens including ***B. anthracis*** and ***F. tularensis*** must be handled under a biohazard safety cabinet to avoid transmission to laboratory staff. Although ***Y. pestis*** is not often transmitted between humans, it is considered a high-risk-level organism due to its ability to cause serious disease.

Various virulence factors allow these organisms to invade and spread within host cells, creating the potential to cause widespread, serious disease. ***B. anthracis, F. tularensis***, and ***Y. pestis*** are all encapsulated with a lipopolysaccharide outer membrane that aids in invasion into host cells and protects bacteria by preventing host-mediated phagocytosis. Both ***F. tularensis*** and ***Y. pestis*** have pili that aid in adhesion to host cells, which is vital to the survival of bacteria in hosts. ***B. anthracis*** has three exotoxins, referred to as the anthrax toxin, that work in unison to bind to, enter, and destroy hosts cells: 3-protective antigen, edema factor, and lethal factor. The anthrax toxin is pertinent for the establishment and spread of disease. ***F. tularensis*** contains acid phosphatase and sidersomes that prevent phagocytosis and sequester host cell iron, respectively. Virulence factors of ***Y. pestis*** include plasminogen activator and fibrinolysin, which prevent phagosome opsonization and are cytotoxic to host cells.

ROLES OF LABORATORY RESPONSE NETWORK AND REGIONAL LABORATORIES REGARDING AGENTS OF BIOTERRORISM

Established by the Centers for Disease Control and Prevention, the **Laboratory Response Network** is a group of laboratories capable of properly responding to biological and chemical threats and other public health emergencies. The Laboratory Response Network is composed of labs from the following sectors: federal, state and local public health, military, food testing, veterinary, environmental, and international. This network allows for the best preparedness and response to biological and chemical terrorism.

Samples suspected of containing biological toxins or microbiological agents that threaten public health are most commonly found or recognized at sentinel laboratories. A **sentinel laboratory** is the foundation of the Laboratory Response Network and is defined as any laboratory capable of detecting and referring chemical or microbial agents. The most common sentinel laboratories include critical access and larger hospital, environmental, food testing, and veterinary labs. Once a threatening agent is recognized and all other organisms have been ruled out, samples are referred to state or local public reference laboratories for confirmation testing. Upon confirmation, regional and public health laboratories are responsible for reporting and referring confirmed bioterrorism agents to the CDC for sample characterization and further investigation.

Analytic Procedures—Mycology, Mycobacteriology, Parasitology, and Virology

MYCOBACTERIUM AND NOCARDIA SPECIES TESTING

Mycobacterium and *Nocardia* species of bacteria are capable of causing a variety of disease states including pulmonary infections and infections of the subcutaneous tissue. The most common specimen collected for pulmonary infections due to these bacteria is **sputum**. First morning sputum samples collected on three consecutive days are ideal for detecting infections caused by these bacteria. **Bronchial** or **gastric washings**, **urine**, and **tissue** samples are also acceptable for *Mycobacterium* and *Nocardia* species recovery. All specimens suspected of such infections should be collected aseptically into sterile, tight-capped containers and transported to the lab as soon as possible. Urine and gastric samples may be refrigerated prior to testing, if needed, to neutralize their acidity.

ACID-FAST REACTION, GROWTH PATTERNS, AND COLONY MORPHOLOGY FOR MYCOBACTERIUM AND NOCARDIA SPECIES TESTING

Listed below are the acid-fast reaction, growth patterns, and colony morphology characteristics of *Mycobacterium* and *Nocardia* species on Löwenstein–Jensen culture media:

- *M. tuberculosis*
    - **Acid-fast:** positive, bright red
    - **Growth pattern:** obligate aerobe, enhanced growth in 5–10% CO_2, visible growth after 3–6 weeks of incubation
    - **Colony morphology:** off white to buff, dry, rough, raised, and wrinkled
- *M. leprae*
    - **Acid-fast:** positive, bright red
    - Growth pattern and colony morphology: cannot be cultivated in vitro
- *M. avium*
    - **Acid-fast:** positive, bright red
    - **Growth pattern:** aerobe, enhanced growth in 5–10% CO_2, visible growth after 3–6 weeks of incubation
    - Colony morphology: buff and smooth
- *Nocardia* species
    - **Acid-fast:** partial, pink, filamentous morphology with branching
    - **Growth pattern:** aerobe, enhanced growth in 5–10% CO_2, visible growth after 3–10 days of incubation
    - **Colony morphology:** yellow to orange, waxy, bumpy, or velvety, with downy aerial hyphae.

MYCOBACTERIUM AND NOCARDIA PATHOGENS

Mycobacteria and *Nocardia* infections occur in immunocompromised patients. These bacteria are opportunistic pathogens that occur naturally in soil, water, and the following sources: **M. tuberculosis**, dust, carpets, clothes, unpasteurized milk; **M. leprae**, human peripheral nerves; **M. avium**, food; and **Nocardia**, normal human oral flora. The pathogen transmission, clinical presentation, and epidemiology are described below:

- **M. tuberculosis** infects approximately one-third of the world's population via respiratory droplet inhalation. Although many patients remain asymptomatic, immunocompromised patients with active tuberculosis exhibit the following symptoms: fever, weight loss, night sweats, weakness, chest pains, and a cough producing sputum and blood. Infections present in three stages: **primary**, active inflammation and granuloma formation that resolves; **latent**, residual bacteria exist in the body; and **postprimary**, dormant bacteria reactivate in the upper lobes of the lungs.
- **M. leprae** causes Hansen's disease, or leprosy, to the skin, mucous membranes, and nerves of those infected. Leprosy is transmittable via inhalation of bacteria or contact with exudates of lesions. Although *M. leprae* has low pathogenicity, clinical manifestations of the disease may become severe and appear after 6 months to more than 40 years of incubation.
- **M. avium** is transmittable through inhalation or consumption of contaminants and is not infectious to most. In severely immunocompromised hosts, *M. avium* causes lymphadenitis or pulmonary and disseminated disease.
- **Nocardia asteroides** and **N. brasiliensis** cause nocardiosis. Infections to healthy hosts occur as skin abscesses, cellulitis, or lymphocutaneous via traumatic inoculation of subcutaneous tissues. Bacterial inhalation causes progressive pneumonia and disseminated disease in immunocompromised patients.

DETECTION OF MYCOBACTERIUM AND NOCARDIA SPECIES

Direct detection methods of *Mycobacterium* and *Nocardia* organisms include microscopic examination with specialized stains and molecular methodologies. Acid-fast stains for clinical specimens colorize bacteria based on the presence or absence of mycolic acid in the bacterial cell wall. **Ziehl–Neelsen** and **Kinyoun** stains are used to observe acid-fast bacteria using a light microscope, whereas **auramine-rhodamine** stain requires a fluorescent microscope. Samples containing mycobacteria will show bright-red bacilli using Ziehl–Neelsen and Kinyoun stains and will fluoresce a yellow to orange color when stained with auramine-rhodamine. The microscopic observation of acid-fast bacilli in any number is considered significant and requires further workup. **Nucleic acid probe** methods can be used to detect the presence of *M. tuberculosis* and *M. avium* genetic material in bacterial colonies grown on culture media. Molecular detection of *M. tuberculosis* directly from clinical specimens can be achieved by using **nucleic acid amplification testing** methods.

DIRECT DETECTION BY MOLECULAR METHODS

Mycobacteria organisms are slow growing and can take between three and eight weeks to cultivate on culture media, which delays patient treatment, or they are unable to be cultivated in the laboratory. Nucleic acid amplification techniques have been developed to detect genetic material from *M. tuberculosis* directly from clinical specimens, in order to provide prompt treatment for patients positive for infection. Ribosomal RNA sequences specific to the *M. tuberculosis* complex are denatured, annealed to oligonucleotide primer probes, and amplified attached to chemiluminescent labeled probes for direct detection.

Biochemically, *Nocardia* species are almost indistinguishable from one another. Molecular methods have been established to aid in identifying pathogenic *Nocardia* past the genus level and to the species level. The 16S ribosomal RNA gene sequencing method amplifies variable regions on the bacterial genome to identify organisms at the species level. Organism identification can be achieved by coupling gene sequencing techniques with PCR methods. PCR-facilitated restriction endonuclease amplification allows for the detection of the following *Nocardia* specific proteins and genes: 65-kDa heat shock protein, essential secretory protein A (secA1), and gyrase B (gyrB).

ANTIMICROBIAL THERAPY

Mycobacteria infections are treated over an extended period of time with combinations of antimicrobial substances due to the high prevalence of varied antibiotic resistance in various species. *M. tuberculosis* infections are treated with a combination of two or three antibiotics over a duration of 6–18 months. The drugs of choice for treating TB are a macrolide, followed by rifampin and ethambutol. Nontuberculous *Mycobacteria* infections are commonly treated over a 6-month to 1-year time period, with a combination of rifampin and ethambutol antibiotics.

The antibiotics of choice for treating infections caused by *Nocardia* species are sulfonamide drugs. Treatment may last from 6–12 months to ensure the eradication of disease-causing organisms. Systemic nocardiosis often requires a combination treatment of a sulfonamide agent and one of the following primary agents: amikacin, ceftriaxone, cefotaxime, linezolid, or imipenem. Erythromycin and third-generation cephalosporin drugs should not be used to treat these infections because *Nocardia* species are known to express antimicrobial resistance to the drugs.

VIRULENCE MECHANISMS
MYCOBACTERIA

The main virulence of all *Mycobacteria* organisms is their mycolic acid cell wall. The waxy nature of the cell wall protects the organism from host defenses and the actions of antibiotics. *Mycobacterium*'s distinct cell wall also causes granuloma formation and induces necrosis following adhesion to host cells. Lipoarabinomannan on the surface of *M. tuberculosis* cells aids in adhesion to host cells while inhibiting host interferon-mediated activity and cytokine production and release and suppressing the proliferation of T lymphocytes, aiding in organism survival. Enzymes and proteins released by the ESX-1-secretion system of *M. tuberculosis* prevent host phagosome-lysosome fusion and evade phagocytosis. *M. tuberculosis* spreads from human to human via the inhalation of infected respiratory droplets, causing primary TB in the lungs that may disseminate and spread throughout the body.

Nontuberculous *Mycobacteria* species are naturally occurring environmental organisms found in soil, dust, and municipal and natural water sources. These opportunistic pathogens often cause symptoms in immunocompromised patients or those with preexisting lung diseases. Lung, skin, and lymph node infections caused by nontuberculous *Mycobacteria* are commonly introduced into the body via prosthetic medical devices. The ability for nontuberculous *Mycobacteria* species to form a biofilm and adhere to surfaces aids in their pathogenicity.

NOCARDIA

Nocardia species naturally occur in soil and water and are responsible for the decomposition of plant material. Humans become infected with *Nocardia* through inhalation or traumatic inoculation during an injury. Skin infections caused by *Nocardia* species present as a skin abscess or cellulitis, lymphocutaneous infections, or a mycetoma infection of the subcutaneous tissue. Pulmonary and disseminated nocardiosis occur following the inhalation of *Nocardia* organisms and often affect immunocompromised hosts. The virulence of *Nocardia* species is dependent on the organisms' stage of growth at the time of inoculation; however, organisms consistently resist phagocytosis by inhibiting phagosome-lysosome fusion and producing a large amount of catalase and hemolysins.

VIROLOGY TESTING

Virology samples should be collected as soon as possible after a patient begins to exhibit signs and symptoms of an infection due to a viral agent. Specimens from various sources and in a variety of transport or preservation media can be submitted for testing. Acceptable specimen sources and special requirements that allow for viral testing are described below:

- **Respiratory specimens**:
    - Nasopharyngeal and throat swabs: easily accessible, acceptable but often contaminated with normal oral flora organisms
    - Nasopharyngeal aspirates: improved recovery of viruses versus nasopharyngeal and throat swabs
    - Bronchial lavages and washings: ideal for detection of lower respiratory tract viruses.
- **Stool or rectal swabs**: detection of enteric viruses including rotavirus and adenovirus, stool preferred over swabs.
- **Urine**: low numbers of certain viruses are detectable; requires three separate first-morning-void, clean-catch specimens up to 10 mL each. Centrifugation and pH neutralization of urine are recommended prior to testing to avoid bacterial and pH contamination.
- **Sterile body fluids and tissues:** sent to the laboratory in sterile containers with a secure lid.
- **Fluid or cells from skin or cervical lesions collected on a swab:** require transport media to maintain viral integrity. Transport media contain antibiotics to avoid bacterial growth and contamination, and they contain fetal calf serum or albumin as a source of nutrients.

PARASITOLOGY

SPECIMENS AND PRESERVATION METHODS FOR PARASITOLOGY TESTING

Stool is the most common parasite specimen collected. Samples must be collected into a clean, dry container with a secure lid, and they must not be contaminated by urine, water, or enemas. Contamination from urine has the ability to destroy motile organisms, water may contain free living organisms, and protozoa may not be detectable for 5–10 days following the administration of barium enemas. Recovery of parasites may be hindered up to 2 weeks after the cessation of certain antibiotics. The most concentrated, early morning and first-void **sputum** and **urine** specimens are collected into dry, sterile containers with a secure lid. **Genital swabs** submitted for parasitic detection require saline to keep them moist for optimal organism recovery. **Skin** and **tissue** samples are best submitted to the laboratory in dry, sterile containers with a secure lid. Fresh **blood** from a fingerstick is the preferred sample for thick and thin blood smear preparations; however, blood collection via venipuncture into an EDTA tube is also acceptable.

Methods of sample storage and preservation based on the type of parasite suspected are as follows:

- **Refrigeration:** eggs, larvae, and amoebic cysts. If amoebic trophozoites are suspected, do not refrigerate.
- 10% formalin and merthiolate-iodine-formalin: eggs, larvae, and amoebic cysts.
- **Polyvinyl alcohol (PVA):** amoebic trophozoites; stained specimen slides can be permanently preserved using this method.

- **Sodium acetate-acetic acid-formalin:** amoebic trophozoites; an environmentally safer alternative to PVA.
- **Schaudinn's fluid:** trophs and cysts, fixative for fresh stool samples.

PATHOGENIC HELMINTHS

Parasitic worms occur naturally in soil. The route of transmission, epidemiology, and disease states associated with helminths are described below:

- **Large intestinal roundworm**, *Ascaris lumbricoides*
  - **Transmission:** fecal–oral route
  - **Epidemiology:** tropical climate and poor sanitation
  - Life cycle:
    - ❖ Eggs hatch in the duodenum and penetrate the intestinal wall.
    - ❖ Adults live and reproduce in the small intestine.
    - ❖ Eggs are passed in feces remain active in soil for 2–6 weeks.
  - **Disease:** intestinal obstruction and pneumonitis caused by larvae migration to lungs
- **Pinworm,** *Enterobius vermicularis*
  - **Transmission:** fecal–oral route
  - **Epidemiology:** school-age children
  - Life cycle:
    - ❖ Adult female matures in the small intestine, incubating for 1–2 months.
    - ❖ Migrates to colon, lays eggs around the anus at night.
    - ❖ Reinfection and infecting others are possible by contact as long as eggs are laid.
  - **Disease:** itchy anal region and associated secondary bacterial infection
- **Whipworm,** *Trichuris trichiura*
  - **Transmission:** fecal–oral route
  - **Epidemiology:** tropical climate and poor sanitation
  - Life cycle:
    - ❖ Eggs hatch in the small intestine.
    - ❖ Adult worms live and reproduce in the large intestine for 3 months after ingestion.
  - **Disease:** bloody, mucous diarrhea and prolapsed rectum in heavy infection
- **New World hookworm,** *Necator americanus,* and **Old World hookworm,** *Ancylostoma duodenale*
  - **Transmission:** skin penetration
  - **Epidemiology:** worldwide distribution
  - Life cycle:
    - ❖ Larvae move to the lungs via the venous system; they are coughed up and swallowed.
    - ❖ Adult worms live and reproduce attached to the small intestinal wall.
  - **Disease:** life cycle-associated
    - ❖ Cutaneous — allergic reactions or "ground itch"
    - ❖ Pulmonary — pneumonitis
    - ❖ Intestinal — anemia and protein deficiency from blood loss at the attachment site.

BLOOD AND TISSUE MICROFILARIAE AND NEMATODE PATHOGENS

The etiology, epidemiology, transmission, and diseases of blood and tissue nematodes and microfilariae are described below:

- **Pork worm,** Trichinella spiralis
  - **Transmission:** Ingesting larvae in undercooked pork.
  - **Etiology and epidemiology:** Worldwide, rural areas, survival requires a host: rodents, domestic pigs, wild boars, other mammals.
  - Life cycle:
    - ❖ Encysted larvae are ingested, and they mature over several weeks in the small intestine.
    - ❖ Adults produce larvae that migrate through tissues and muscle.
  - **Disease:** resembles food poisoning, muscle cell destruction, eosinophilia, possible myocardial involvement.
  - **Microfilariae,** early life stage nematodes — an arthropod intermediate host is required. Vectors introduce third-stage filarial larvae that penetrate into human skin via bite wounds during blood feedings.
- *Wuchereria bancrofti*
  - **Vector:** Anopheles, *Culex* mosquitoes
  - Epidemiology: Worldwide
  - Life cycle:
    - ❖ Adults live and reproduce in the lymphatic system.
    - ❖ Microfilariae migrate through lymph and blood channels.
  - **Disease:** elephantiasis — permanent lymphatic blockage, genitalia and lower extremities
- **Eye worm,** *Loa Loa*
  - **Vector:** Chrysops (deer) fly
  - **Epidemiology:** West and Central Africa
  - Life cycle:
    - ❖ Adults live and reproduce in subcutaneous tissues.
    - ❖ Microfilariae in peripheral blood during the day and the lungs at night.
  - **Disease:** "caliber swelling" — localized swelling, with itching on arms, legs, and near joints; blindness
- *Onchocerca volvulus*
  - **Vector:** Simulium (black) fly
  - **Epidemiology:** "river blindness" leading cause of blindness in Africa
  - Life cycle:
    - ❖ Adults live and reproduce in subcutaneous connective tissue for 10–15 years.
    - ❖ Microfilariae in the skin and connective tissues lymphatics.
  - **Disease:** severe dermatitis, blindness, onchocercoma — nodule containing an encapsulated adult.

CESTODE PARASITIC PATHOGENS

The etiology, epidemiology, transmission, and diseases of tapeworms are described below:

- **Beef tapeworm**, *Taenia saginata*
  - **Transmission:** ingestion of larvae in undercooked beef
  - **Etiology and epidemiology:** common in Eastern Europe, Russia, Eastern Africa, and Latin America; poor sanitation; free-ranging cattle
  - Life cycle:
    - ❖ Eggs enter the environment by infected human feces.
    - ❖ Livestock eat vegetation with eggs that migrate to striated muscle and become cysticerci, where they can be ingested by humans in undercooked meat.
    - ❖ Cysticerci attach to the small intestine.
  - **Disease:** taeniasis — abdominal pain, loss of appetite, weight loss
- **Pork tapeworm**, *Taenia solium*
  - **Transmission:** ingestion of larvae in undercooked pork
  - **Etiology and epidemiology:** highest infection rates are in Latin America, Asia, and Africa; poor sanitation; free-ranging pigs
  - **Life cycle:** the same as *T. saginata*
  - **Disease:** cysticercosis — rare, larval cysts in the brain and muscles, causing seizures
- **Dwarf tapeworm**, *Hymenolepis nana*
  - **Transmission:** ingestion of eggs
  - **Etiology and epidemiology:** the most common tapeworm in the US
  - Life cycle:
    - ❖ Eggs passed in human feces survive for 10 days in the environment.
    - ❖ Eggs are ingested by a beetle or flea intermediate host and develop into cysticercoids that are ingested by humans or rodents.
    - ❖ Adults mature, reside, and reproduce in the small intestine.
  - **Disease:** most asymptomatic, heavy infections are due to autoinfection — weakness, headache, abdominal pain, diarrhea, anorexia.

TREMATODE AND PROTOZOA PARASITIC PATHOGENS

Pathogenic parasite etiology, epidemiology, transmission, and diseases are described below:

- *Schistosomes*, blood flukes
  - **Transmission:** free-swimming cercariae are released from the snail into the water and penetrate the skin
  - **Etiology and epidemiology:** found in the Western Hemisphere, not the US — snail host not present
  - Disease:
    - ❖ "Swimmer's itch" — dermatitis
    - ❖ Eosinophilia, bloody urine and diarrhea
    - ❖ Progressive chronic inflammatory disease involving the liver, intestines, and bladder
- *Entamoeba histolytica*
  - **Transmission:** fecal–oral, ingestion of contaminated food or water
  - **Etiology and epidemiology:** most common in tropical climates and poor sanitation
  - **Disease:** amebiasis — intestinal tract ulcers, liver and lung abscesses

- *Giardia lamblia*
  - o **Transmission:** fecal–oral; ingestion of contaminated drinking or recreational water is the most common mode of transmission
  - o **Etiology and epidemiology:** distributed worldwide in water, soil food, or on surfaces; common in daycare centers and in acquired immunodeficiency syndrome (AIDS) patients
  - o **Disease:** giardiasis-diarrhea, duodenitis, malabsorption of fats
- *Plasmodium* **species**
  - o **Transmission:** bloodstream inoculated via bite of female *Anopheles* mosquito
  - o **Etiology and epidemiology:** most associated with low altitude, tropical and subtropical climates. *P. falciparum* — predominant species worldwide
  - o **Disease:** nonspecific symptoms — fever, chills, headache, myalgia, weakness, vomiting, diarrhea, splenomegaly, anemia, hypoglycemia, pulmonary or renal dysfunction, neurologic changes
    - ❖ *P. vivax* — benign tertian
    - ❖ *P. ovale* — tertian malaria
    - ❖ *P. falciparum* — malignant tertian malaria, blackwater fever
    - ❖ *P. malariae* — quartan malaria.
- *Babesia microti*
  - o **Transmission:** bloodstream inoculated via deer tick bite or transmitted during blood transfusions
  - o **Etiology and epidemiology:** most common in the Northeastern and Upper Midwestern US; no geographical limit on transmission via blood transfusion
  - o **Disease:** babesiosis — fever, fatigue, myalgia, GI symptoms, dark urine, mild splenomegaly or hepatomegaly, jaundice.

PROTOZOA PARASITIC PATHOGENS

The etiology, epidemiology, transmission, and diseases of protozoa are described below:

- *Trypanosoma cruzi*
  - o **Transmission**: feces of an infected "kissing bug" is scratched or rubbed into its bite wound on humans, also transmittable by blood transfusion
  - o **Etiology and epidemiology:** North and South America, mainly rural Latin America
  - o **Disease:** Chagas' disease
    - ❖ **Acute** — asymptomatic or mild fever and swelling around the inoculation site
    - ❖ **Chronic** — arrhythmias, poorly pumping heart, dilated esophagus or colon causing issues eating or passing stool
- *Leishmania*
  - o **Transmission:** released into human via bite of infected sandfly
  - o **Etiology and epidemiology:** New World disease found in Asia, the Middle East, Africa, and Southern Europe. Old World disease found in Mexico and Central and South America. It does not occur in Australia, the Pacific Islands, Chile, or Uruguay.
  - o **Disease:** cutaneous leishmaniasis
    - ❖ *L. donovani* — visceral leishmaniasis (kala-azar), fever, weight loss, hepatosplenomegaly
    - ❖ *L. tropica* — Old World cutaneous leishmaniasis, also known as Oriental sore, skin sores

71

> ❖ **L. braziliensis** — New World cutaneous or mucocutaneous; sores in the nose, mouth, or throat

- ***Cryptosporidium parvum***
  - **Transmission:** fecal–oral, ingestion of contaminated drinking or recreational water is the most common mode of transmission
  - **Etiology and epidemiology:** most common cause of waterborne disease in the US
  - **Disease:** Cryptosporidiosis
    - ❖ **Immunocompetent host** — asymptomatic or self-limiting, watery diarrhea, vomiting, abdominal cramps
    - ❖ **Immunocompromised host** — symptoms listed above, severe diarrhea, can also affect other parts of the GI tract or the respiratory tract.

MICROSCOPIC OBSERVATION AND IDENTIFICATION OF PARASITES

Ova and parasites are identified microscopically by key characteristics using a variety of stains and slide preparations. Fresh samples can be observed as a **wet mount**, mixed with saline to observe motility and iodine to kill trophozoites and enhance nuclear material. Fresh and preserved specimens can be permanently stained for the detection, identification, quantification, and permanent recording of parasites. The **trichrome** stain is the most common stain used for identifying intestinal parasites. It is rapid and simple, and it yields uniformly stained parasites, yeast, human cells, and artifacts. Cysts, trophozoites, and small protozoa undetected on wet mount can be identified with trichrome stains. The **modified trichrome** stain is diagnostic for detecting unicellular, intracellular microsporidian parasites. Blood smears stained with **Wright** and **Giemsa** stains provide rapid detection of malarial parasite rings in RBCs. **Acid-fast** staining identifies coccidian oocysts that are difficult to detect with other stains, and it is diagnostic for *Cryptosporidium, Isospora*, and *Cyclospora* species. Intestinal parasites can be quantified and their microfilarial sheath can be observed by staining with **iron hematoxylin**.

Key microscopic characteristics evaluated for helminth eggs and other parasite identification include:

- **Shape**: oval, round, ellipse, symmetrical, elongated, lightbulb or barrel shaped
- **Size**: measured in microns
- **Color:** colorless, yellow, brown
- **Texture, outer shell appearance:** operculated, smooth, scalloped edge, lateral or terminal spine, polar or bipolar filaments.

If recovered, adult worms can be observed for key identifying features including flat or round body shape, pointed or notched tails, the shape and number of teeth, sheath, and the presence and arrangement of nuclei on the tail.

MACROSCOPIC IDENTIFICATION

Ova, cyst, and parasite examinations begin with the evaluation of macroscopic properties of the sample. Characteristics including the consistency, color, and presence of certain substances indicate the presence of a parasitic infection and provide information toward obtaining a positive parasite identification.

The **consistency** of a stool specimen can indicate which form of a parasite will exist in the specimen. Helminth eggs may be present in stool of any consistency, whereas formed stools contain protozoan cysts, soft stools contain trophozoites or cysts, and liquid stool samples will contain trophozoites. Stool can be macroscopically examined for the presence of **mucus, blood,** or

macroscopic parasites. The **color** of stool samples can also provide insight to the presence of parasitic infections. Black stools indicate the presence of iron or blood, and light-tan or white stool samples indicate barium or the absence of bile, all of which indicate the presence of parasites in the gastrointestinal tract.

DIRECT AND MOLECULAR TECHNIQUES TO DETECT PARASITIC INFECTIONS

Microscopy examination of permanently stained specimen slides is the most common and most widely used direct technique for detecting parasites. Large parasites or adult worms can be recovered and visually inspected for identification. Pinworm infections can be detected by using a paddle for collecting a sample from the perianal region. The sticky portion of the paddle is gently pressed against the skin surrounding the rectum three to four times. Samples are collected first thing in the morning because adult female pinworms lay eggs in this area each night. The **pinworm prep** paddle is visually observed for the presence of pinworm eggs, which would diagnose an infection.

Other methods for the detection of parasites have been developed for the determination of parasitic infections. Rapid tests kits use **enzyme immunoassay** and **immunofluorescent assay** methodologies to detect antigens produced as a result of parasites in the body. Enzyme immunoassay methods detect parasitic antigens with parasite-specific monoclonal antibodies, and immunofluorescent assay tests use the same methodology with the addition of fluorescent dyes to represent the antigen–antibody complexes formed. **Real-time PCR** and **multiplex PCR** methods are used to detect molecular material of ova and parasites in specimens. Multiplex assays allow for the detection of many different parasites at the same time and use a single sample. Molecular multiplex methods use a variety of molecular primers to target gene sequences of multiple organisms.

MYCOLOGY
SPECIMENS FOR MYCOLOGY TESTING

Cultures for fungal organisms can be set up from samples of any tissue or body fluid including hair, skin, nails, tissue, sputum, urine, blood, bone marrow, CSF, and other normally sterile body fluids. Samples must be collected in screw-cap tubes or tape plates to avoid accidental opening, spilling, and drying of specimens in transport. Swabbed samples are acceptable for culture but are the least desirable transport system due to the increased drying and contamination potential. All mycology samples should be transported to the lab as soon as possible for the best chance of recovering organisms. Specimens remain the most viable when held at room temperature and should be saved for at least 6 weeks because fungi grow slowly.

MYCOLOGY PATHOGENS

Found worldwide, fungi are naturally occurring organisms that are able to cause infection when they enter the lungs by inhalation or when they enter the tissues by trauma. Some species of fungi are part of the human normal flora that cause opportunistic infections in immunocompromised hosts. Hosts most susceptible to fungal infections include premature babies and neonates, HIV/AIDS patients, and those taking an immunosuppressant drug.

Candida normally live as commensal organisms on the skin and in the mouth, throat, GI tract, and vagina. *C. albicans,* the most common species to cause infection, causes thrush infections in the throat or mouth and yeast infections of the skin, genitals, and blood. *C. auris* is associated with hospital outbreaks and is considered a rising pathogen due to its multidrug-resistant nature.

Cryptococcus neoformans is found in soil and in pigeon and other bird feces. Inhalation of fungi from the environment causes a pneumonia-like illness, with meningitis and encephalitis occurring in severely immunocompromised patients.

Aspergillus spores inhaled from the air cause aspergillosis, which presents as allergic reactions and lung, cutaneous, or invasive infections. *A. fumigatus* is the most common pathogenic species, followed by *A. flavus*, which often affects agriculturists with farmer's lung.

Histoplasma capsulatum occurs in soil and in bird and bat feces and causes histoplasmosis when inhaled. Symptoms range from mild: fever, head and muscle aches, dry cough, and fatigue; to chronic: mimics tuberculosis symptoms; to disseminated: fatal if left untreated.

Pneumocystis jiroveci causes atypical interstitial plasma-cell pneumonia when respiratory droplets of an infected human or other mammal are inhaled.

YEAST IDENTIFICATIONS

The results of **biochemical reactions** of yeast isolates are used to differentiate major pathogens from one another. *Candida albicans*, the most common pathogenic yeast, and *Cryptococcus neoformans*, a potentially fatal pathogen, can be differentiated from one another based on their urease test reactions, with *C. albicans* presenting as urease negative and *C. neoformans* reacting as urease positive.

Automated methods for the identification of pathogenic yeast species aid in providing rapid and confident determination of major pathogens. These methods use a panel or test card loaded with chemicals with the specific purpose of differentiating yeast species from one another. Biochemical reactions obtained from a specimen or culture isolate are compared to an information database within automated systems. The database compares biochemical patterns and potential pattern variations of known yeast species to those obtained from the unknown isolate to determine its identification. Automated methods can obtain an organism identification in as little as 4 hours, allowing for the rapid diagnosis and treatment of yeast infections.

MALDI-TOF MS allows for early identification and disease diagnosis of fungal infections in a fast and precise manner. Yeast species can be identified by MALDI-TOF MS even in a mixed-colony culture by matching unique specimen reactions to computer database records of known yeast species.

FUNGAL PATHOGENS

Most fungal species are often first identified by Gram stain procedures or microscopic examination of urine sediment. In a **Gram stain**, yeast will appear as budding cells or pseudohyphae pigmented purple or a blue-black color. Preparing hair, skin, or nail samples with **potassium hydroxide (KOH)** on a slide with a coverslip allows for nonfungal cells and debris to be cleared and makes fungal elements more easily visible. KOH-prepared slides can be stained with **Calcofluor-white** stain and viewed under a fluorescent microscope. Fungal elements are detected by fluorescing on a black background in a blue-white or bright-green color, depending on the microscope filters used. **India ink** is added to centrifuged sediment of CSF samples for the rapid detection of *C. neoformans*. If present, encapsulated *C. neoformans* buds will appear on a black background with a large clear area around them. Filamentous and branching *Nocardia* species can be differentiated from other actinomycetes with the **acid-fast** stain. **Gömöri's methenamine silver** stain aids in the detection of *P. jiroveci* by staining carbohydrates in the organisms' cell walls black to brown colors.

Key characteristics of detecting and identifying fungal pathogens microscopically include:

- Intracellular or extracellular
- Shape: budding, pseudohyphae, hyphae, filamentous
- Encapsulated or no capsule present

Examples of microscopic morphology of pathogens are as follows:

- **Candida species:** yeast with pseudohyphae
- **C. albicans:** small, extracellular yeast buds and pseudohyphae
- **C. neoformans:** encapsulated yeast, no pseudohyphae
- **Histoplasma capsulatum:** very small, intracellular yeast in tissue samples.

SELECTIVE CULTURE MEDIA AND GERM TUBE TEST TO IDENTIFY MYCOLOGICAL PATHOGENS

Many fungal species are fastidious organisms that require certain nutrients to grow. Fungi are also slow growing on culture media and require bactericidal antibiotics to avoid bacterial overgrowth and increase fungal recovery. The following culture media are used in identifying fungal pathogens:

- **Sabouraud agar:** for the recovery of dermatophytes from cutaneous samples and yeast from vaginal cultures
- **Sabouraud heart infusion agar:** for the primary recovery and isolation of fastidious saprophytic and dimorphic fungi
- **Sabouraud dextrose agar:** subculture recovered fungi to enhance sporulation and provides more characteristic colony morphology for identification
- **Mycobiotic agar:** comprised of Sabouraud dextrose agar with added antibiotics for the primary recovery of dermatophytes
  - Cycloheximide: inhibits saprophytic and nonpathogenic fungi
  - Chloramphenicol: inhibits bacterial growth added
- **Czapek's agar**: to subculture *Aspergillus* fungi for species differentiation
- **Niger seed agar**: for *C. neoformans* identification.

The **germ tube test** is a simple, rapid test for *C. albicans* identification. The procedure is based on the species' ability to produce germ tubes from their yeast cells. An amount of 0.5 mL of sheep or rabbit serum and a yeast colony are added to a test tube and incubated for 2–3 hours at 35–37 °C. Following incubation, a drop of the serum suspension is added to a microscope slide with a coverslip and observed microscopically under low power. The presence of germ tubes extending from yeast cells indicate *C. albicans.* Germ tubes are hypha-like extensions of yeast cells with no constrictions at the point where the extension originates.

COLONY MORPHOLOGY AND GROWTH CHARACTERISTICS OF MAJOR PATHOGENS

Sabouraud dextrose agar (SDA) is the culture media used for the cultivation of yeasts and molds with a pH of 5.6 to optimize the growth of fungal pathogens. Antibiotics can be added to the medium to inhibit bacterial overgrowth. Due to the slow-growing nature of many fungi, mycological cultures are often kept for four to six weeks to properly assess growth. Listed below are the major human mycological pathogens, with their growth requirements and colony morphology:

C. albicans

- **SDA:** cream-colored, smooth colonies with a yeast-like odor after 24–48 hours of incubation at 25–37 °C
- **Blood agar:** white, creamy colonies with foot-like projections around the margin
- **CHROMagar:** green-colored colonies

C. neoformans

- **SDA**: white to cream-colored, smooth, mucoid colonies after 48–72 hours of incubation at 37 °C in 5% CO_2
- **Bird seed agar:** brown-pigmented colonies

A. fumigatus

- **SDA:** blue-green, velvety or powdery colonies with a narrow white margin on the front of the medium and a pale-yellow color on the back of the medium after 72 hours of incubation at 25–45 °C

H. capsulatum

- **SDA:** white, fluffy mold within five days of incubation at 25–37 °C. Colonies turn a buff to brown color as they age. Incubation at 37 °C may produce cream-colored, wrinkled, moist, yeast-like colonies.

MANUAL AND AUTOMATED IDENTIFICATION METHODS

Major yeast and fungus pathogens are differentiated from one another based on their specific biochemical reactions. Biochemical reactions for the identification of pathogens can be performed manually by microbiologists, or they can be performed by sophisticated automated systems. Automated systems are able to differentiate and identify organisms by performing various biochemical reactions on a single test card or panel. A solution is prepared with sterile liquid and an organism inoculated from a culture plate. The inoculate dilution is added to the test card, which has differentiating chemicals loaded into individual test wells. Automated systems compare the pattern of biochemical reactions produced by an isolate to a computerized database for proper identification of the organism. Some organisms may be identified by automated systems within 4 hours; however, most isolates are determined within 12–24 hours.

Certain biochemical reactions provide a simple technique for the differentiation of major yeast pathogens. For example, the urease test is a quick biochemical reaction that can determine the difference between the most common, and most easily treatable, yeast pathogen, *C. albicans*, and a less common, potentially fatal, yeast species, *C. neoformans*.

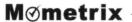

Postanalytic Procedures

PROPER DOCUMENTATION PRACTICES IN LABORATORIES

Good laboratory practices include proper documentation of laboratory operations. Patient results, quality control and calibration values, competency testing, and documentation of troubleshooting are important for monitoring a laboratory's performance and following a continuous quality improvement plan. Accuracy in documenting patient laboratory results is necessary for providing appropriate patient care. Printed or electronic reports allow for physicians to follow up on and review results and are more accurate with less chance of clerical errors than verbal results. Computer interfaces between the analyzers and the LIS provide the documentation of correct patient results in a more efficient manner, with delta checks, or internal warnings of change between an individual patient's previous and current results. Delta checks alert staff to manually review patient results for accuracy and rule out any preanalytical or analytical mishaps. Comprehensive documentation of quality control and calibration results allows for the evaluation of analyzers' functionality and establish trends in analyte analysis.

REPORTING URGENT OR CRITICAL VALUES

Critical or panic values are defined as possibly life-threatening laboratory results that must be acknowledged and communicated to the patient's physician as soon as possible. An automated LIS will flag critical values to alert staff of the need to review and communicate results. Required information while reporting critical values varies among individual labs, but commonly the following information must be documented along with panic laboratory results: the date and time the results were given to the physician; the name of the physician or qualified healthcare professional that the results were relayed to; and the name of the laboratory staff member who reviewed, relayed, and verified the result. Other pertinent information regarding the sample may also be documented, including noting that the sample was inspected for preanalytical or analytical errors or that the testing was repeated to verify the legitimacy of the results.

REVIEWING LABORATORY RESULTS AND THE RESULT AUTOVERIFICATION PROCESS

All laboratory results must be reviewed and approved by staff before they are released to providers. Reviewing the results is necessary for ensuring that laboratory procedures are being followed, the instrumentation is working properly, and that the results reflect the true state of a patient's health status. Providing accurate test results is imperative to the physician's decision-making process for providing appropriate care to patients.

Computer-based algorithms are able to automatically review and verify laboratory results without manual intervention. Laboratories are able to design, customize, implement, and validate autoverification rules based on the needs of their individual patient populations. Autoverification rules and limits are established by rule-based, neural network, or pattern-recognition computer algorithms. Although normal results with minimal variation from pervious results will automatically be released by the system, abnormal results will display flags and will require manual review. Flags for manual review are developed for the following circumstances: critical values, values outside of analyzer limitations, and results failing the checks and balances set up within the system.

ISSUING CORRECTED REPORTS

The process of detecting and correcting inaccurate results that have been mistakenly verified is necessary to assuring appropriate patient diagnosis and care. Once an error is detected, the ordering provider must be promptly notified of the inaccurate result, the error must be corrected, and an accurate result must be provided to the ordering physician. The Clinical Laboratory

Improvement Amendments of 1988 (CLIA '88) regulations mandate that all corrected reports issued are accompanied by a written report of the circumstances leading to the erroneous result, the actions taken to correct the issue, and a proposed plan to address changes in operations that will prevent similar mistakes in the future.

REPORTING RESULTS TO INFECTION CONTROL AND PUBLIC HEALTH DEPARTMENTS

Laboratory results indicating and confirming certain infectious diseases are required to be reported to infection control and public health departments. Results reported to hospital infection control departments are often used in the evaluation of care quality and monitoring hospital versus community-acquired infections. Disease states such as pneumonia or *C. difficile* infections are closely followed by infection prevention departments to ensure that hospital standard operating procedures allow for the optimal environment for patient care. Local and state health departments require the reporting of communicable diseases and pathogens with the potential to cause an outbreak or public health hazard to reduce the morbidity and mortality of diseases. Positive results for sexually transmitted and hepatitis, or *E. coli* 0157 infections, and potential agents of bioterrorism are examples of laboratory tests submitted to public health departments. Patient demographics and contact information are also provided to these departments for their use in evaluating and studying the state of public health and detection of certain outbreaks in the area.

Laboratory Operations

Quality Assessment and Troubleshooting

QUALITY ASSURANCE

Quality assurance is a set of policies, procedures, and practices derived from the consideration of any and all factors that may affect patient care. Laboratory quality assurance programs are necessary for producing reliable test results. These functions are divided into three categories, determined by when they occur in the analysis process.

Preanalytical functions are actions taken before a sample has begun being tested that can affect the patient care process. Examples of preanalytical functions are specimen collection, labeling, transport, and preservation prior to analysis. Quality assurance policies ensure that preanalytical processes allow for proper testing to be performed on correct patient samples.

Analytical functions take place during the testing process itself. Instrument and assay validation, quality control data, and result verification belong to the analytical category of quality assurance. Comprehensive education and training of testing personnel also belong to quality assurance programs. Following quality assurance policies and standards allows for accurate results to be obtained and reported by laboratory professionals.

Postanalytical functions of a quality assurance program occur after the analysis of a specimen. Included in this category is providing proper documentation for a clinical specimen, ensuring that the correct result is being reported to clinical staff, and revealing any actions taken regarding the interpretation of results.

CALIBRATION AND QUALITY CONTROL CHECKS OF INSTRUMENTS

Generally, all instruments used to generate, measure, and assess data should be routinely calibrated and tested, based on standards and standard operating procedures. The frequency may vary, but some require daily **calibration** while others need calibration every few months. Equipment should also be calibrated if mechanical or other problems have occurred. Calibration may be done manually or semi- or completely automatically, and procedures may vary, but usually include:

- Testing calibrators, solutions, or samples with known values, to determine accuracy of measurement.
- Carefully preparing calibrators, including correct volumes.
- Following directions exactly (according to manufacturer's guidelines), maintaining the proper conditions (light, heat, ventilation), and using calibrators in the correct order and manner.
- Noting the need for adjustments to the equipment or process.

Calibration is part of quality control, but those instruments, supplies, or equipment that are not involved in directly generating, measuring, or assessing data generally do not require calibration but are maintained as part of general quality control.

POINT-OF-CARE TESTING (POCT)

Point-of-care testing (**POCT**) is described as diagnostic laboratory testing performed near the patient in settings such as at the patient bedside or in physician offices. The complexity of POCT is determined by assessing the knowledge, training, reagent and material preparation, technique for

79

operation, quality control characteristics, maintenance, troubleshooting, and interpretation required for each method.

Categories of POCT:

- **Waived**: Simple testing procedure with little chance of negative patient outcome IF performed inaccurately, little judgment is required. Any over-the-counter test approved by the FDA. Examples include influenza and rapid strep tests.
- **Moderate complexity**: Typically automated, more complex than waived tests, most laboratory tests are in this category. Examples include blood counts and routine chemistries.
- **High complexity**: Nonautomated assays requiring highly trained personnel and considerable use of judgment. Examples include microbiology procedures and blood bank crossmatches.
- **Provider-performed microscopy**: Subcategory of moderate complexity testing, in-office slide examination of body fluid performed by the physician or provider, e.g., wet mount.

CLIA '88 STANDARDS FOR POCT FACILITIES AND ADVANTAGES OF POCT

POCT testing is regulated, and facilities must be licensed under the Clinical Laboratory Improvement Amendments of 1988 (**CLIA '88**). Federal guidelines require POCT sites to adhere to good laboratory practice standards, comprised of training of personnel, competency evaluations, and quality control performance. State and city governments may enact more strict or specific regulations as they see fit.

POCT is more accessible than traditional laboratory testing methods, requires a smaller sample volume, and has a quicker turnaround time. This increases patient convenience, while acting to reduce lengths of hospital stays and improve care management. The cost of providing POCT and the associated training, competency, and quality standards must be taken into consideration to maintain the provision of appropriate patient care.

COMPLIANCE

Laboratory compliance encompasses policies, practices, and procedures that must be followed to ensure accurate results and good patient care. Regulatory agencies set standards to establish good laboratory practices and provide guidance for clinical laboratories. Compliance with these practices is instrumental in the success of laboratories and the facilities that support them. Failure to follow these practices, or other standards set by governing bodies, can result in events that adversely affect patient outcomes. Noncompliance can be detected through inspections, whistleblower complaints, or unsatisfactory patient events. Recognition and resolution of laboratory noncompliance must be acknowledged and submitted to governing bodies in order for a laboratory to remain in good standing and prove that efforts are being made to support good laboratory practices.

VOLUNTARY ACCREDITING AND MANDATORY REGULATORY AGENCIES AND ACTS FOR LABORATORY OPERATIONS

Mandatory regulatory agencies:

- **Department of Health and Human Services** (DHHS) — oversees the following:
  - **Food and Drug Administration** (FDA) — regulates medical devices and blood products; approves new tests, technology, and instruments for laboratories

- o **Centers for Medicare and Medicaid Services** (CMS) — agency responsible for CLIA '88, Medicare and Medicaid Services
  - o **Office of the Inspector General** (OIG) — part of CMS, laboratories can participate in a voluntary compliance program to prevent fraud and abuse
  - o **Centers for Disease Control and Prevention** (CDC) — develops disease prevention guidelines and standards
- **Department of Transportation** (DOT) — Hazardous Materials Standard requires specific training and procedures for shipping biohazardous materials
- **United States Postal Service** (USPS) — directions for properly packaging biological specimens for shipping
- **Occupational Safety and Health Administration** (OSHA) — employee safety regulations
- **Equal Employment Opportunity Commission** (EEOC) — prohibits job discrimination
- **Health Insurance Portability and Accountability Act** (HIPAA) — protects confidentiality of patients' healthcare information
- **Clinical Laboratory Improvement Act of 1988** (CLIA '88) — standards for laboratory practice and quality to ensure the accuracy of testing

Voluntary Accrediting Agencies: all in accordance with CLIA '88 standards:

- **The Joint Commission** (TJC) — inspects and accredits hospitals and healthcare facilities
- **College of American Pathologists** (CAP) — clinical laboratories
- **Commission for Office Laboratory Accreditation** (COLA) — community hospital and physician office laboratories.

INSPECTIONS, PROFICIENCY TESTING, AND COMPETENCY ASSESSMENT PROGRAMS IN LABORATORIES

Under CLIA '88, all laboratories must be certified every 2 years to continue to prove that they are operating under the appropriate standards for testing. Although the extent of the regulations enforced is determined by the complexity of testing done in a facility, all laboratory testing sites must take part in the following activities:

- Quality assurance and quality control
- Proficiency testing
- Performance improvement
- Personnel qualifications
- Patient test management

Proficiency testing is part of the laboratory's quality assurance program. Unknown test samples are sent to a group of participating labs for testing, and their results are compared to one another. Proficiency testing allows for laboratories to evaluate the accuracy of their procedures, assays, instruments, and personnel.

A **competency assessment** program comprises periodic evaluations of staff and testing personnel. Supervisory staff must review each shift's work for any errors and omissions. Competency assessment provides laboratories with a way to ensure that testing personnel are properly trained and that they are following policies and procedures, and it acknowledges any improvements that can be made for patient and employee safety.

HARDWARE

Computer hardware consists of all of the physical parts of a computer. All machinery and equipment that makes up the computer and its related components are considered hardware. This includes computer disks, cables, the CPU (central processing unit), printers, keyboard, modem, and any other physical parts of the computer. A computer's hardware is what indicates what a computer is capable of doing.

SOFTWARE

Computer software, on the other hand, is all of the programs that tell a computer how to operate. Software can be divided into application software, which are programs that manipulate and process data, and system software, which control the computer and other programs. Software is written in various programming languages, and the software is responsible for controlling what the hardware does and how the hardware operates.

BENEFITS OF COMPUTERIZED DATA AUTOMATION IN THE LABORATORY

Computerized automation of laboratory data has several advantages. For one, with the computer taking care of recording and storing data, laboratory technicians have more time to do other clinical tasks, such as performing laboratory tests. This increases laboratory productivity. Data stored on a computer, instead of paper laboratory reports, requires less storage space and can be encrypted for confidentiality. Another reason that computer automation is beneficial is that with data stored in a computer system, doctors and nurses can access such data much faster than if paper reports had to be mailed or faxed to them. In some cases, doctors can log onto a hospital computer system to see test results right away. And, using a computer to record data leads to fewer filing and billing errors on the part of the laboratory technicians.

MAINTAINING THE SECURITY OF COMPUTERS AND DATABASES

Security of laboratory computers and databases is a very important issue in the medical laboratory. Patient confidentiality must be kept at all times, and patients' data must not get into the wrong hands or be viewed by the wrong set of eyes. Because of this, there are various methods that laboratories can use to keep their computers and databases safe. Using passwords and identification numbers or names for each laboratory technician or doctor is a widely used method for security. Also, limiting the access to the computers can help as well. Using voice recognition technologies or keys that must be inserted into locks on the computers can keep computers and data safe. Various software programs, such as anti-virus, anti-spyware, and encryption software can enhance security. It must be noted, however, that security measures should not greatly impact the ease of using the computers.

> **Review Video: Ethics and Confidentiality in Counseling**
> Visit mometrix.com/academy and enter code: 250384

Safety

LABORATORY'S RESPONSIBILITY IN PREVENTING INFECTIONS DUE TO BLOODBORNE PATHOGENS

OSHA requires laboratories to operate following **universal** or **standard precautions**. Such precautions are defined as treating every bodily fluid as potentially infectious or containing bloodborne pathogens. Common bloodborne pathogens are HIV and hepatitis B and C. To protect employees in the event of an accidental exposure, employers must provide hepatitis B vaccinations at no cost to employees in positions with moderate to high risk of exposure.

Laboratories must provide staff with the proper **personal protective equipment**, PPE, for them to perform their jobs safely. PPE minimizes the risk of exposure to potentially infectious samples by providing an extra barrier between samples and the staff's skin or mucous membranes. Additionally, engineered equipment is used to provide protection for laboratory staff from potentially infectious materials.

Common PPE:

- Gloves
- Lab coats
- Safety goggles

Engineered safety equipment:

- Work shields — protection from splashes
- Needle safety devices — protect against needlestick injuries
- Biohazard safety hoods — protection from aerosol-inducing samples.

OSHA

OSHA's acts and standards make up a federally created system put in place to ensure workplace safety. OSHA standards include requirements for warning labels, alerts for potential hazards, appropriate PPE, exposure procedures, and the implementation of proper training and employee education. Laboratories must create, educate, and follow a formal safety program, provide specifically mandated plans for chemical and biohazardous exposure, as well as hygiene standards, and identify various hazards in the workplace.

SAFETY DATA SHEETS (SDS) FOR CHEMICALS AND REAGENTS

Safety data sheets (SDS) exist as the core of OHSA's safety standards. An SDS is required for every chemical present in the laboratory, to provide information regarding its physical and chemical properties, safe handling, proper storage and disposal, and the potential hazards associated. SDS information is provided by chemical manufacturers and suppliers and must accompany each chemical upon shipment.

Information on SDS:

- Trade name
- Chemical name and synonyms
- Chemical family
- Manufacturer's name and address
- Emergency phone number for more info related to the chemical
- Hazardous ingredients
- Physical data
- Fire and explosion data
- Health hazard and protection information
  - Effects of overexposure/exceeding threshold of allowable exposure
  - PPE and equipment requirements
  - First aid practices
  - Spill information and directions
  - Procedures for proper disposal.

OSHA-Mandated Regulations for Occupational Exposure to Bloodborne Pathogens

The OSHA-mandated "Occupational Exposure to Bloodborne Pathogens" standard requires laboratories to create, implement, and comply with plans to ensure laboratory staff safety from potential infectious pathogens. Employees must be educated at least annually on their laboratory's chemical and biohazard waste management and emergency exposure procedures. In the event of an exposure, policies and procedures involving such emergencies must always be available to laboratory staff to safely and properly handle all injuries, materials, and waste products.

Training and Proper Procedures for Packaging and Transporting Category A and Category B Biological Specimens

All laboratory personnel who take part in the packaging and shipment of biohazardous materials must complete a comprehensive training course within 90 days of hire and once every 2 years after that. Proper education and training are pertinent for limiting exposure during transport and providing information on a package's contents if exposure occurs.

Category A: a specimen that is capable of causing a permanent disability or a life-threatening or fatal disease to a healthy individual upon exposure

Category B: a specimen that is not in a form capable of causing a permanent disability or a life-threatening or fatal disease to a healthy individual upon exposure

"Exempt specimen": used only by USPS and the International Air Transport Association, defined as a specimen unlikely to cause disease in humans or animals and with a minimal likelihood of a pathogen being present.

Packaging guidelines for shipping:

- Primary packaging that is leakproof
- Absorbent material if the specimen is not a solid
- Secondary packaging that is also leakproof
- Itemized list of the package contents
- A third, rigid outer layer that is able to withstand a 4-foot drop test without breaking/opening
- Biohazard labeling on the outside of the packaging:
  o Category A — UN2814 Infectious substance, affecting humans
  o Category B — UN3373 Biological substance

Laboratory Mathematics

Significant Figures

Significant figures enable scientists to determine which measurements are very precise and which measurements are not as precise. Every measurement has uncertainty. When recording data, the use of the correct number of significant figures indicates the precision of the equipment being used to measure the data. In general, measurements are recorded only to the first uncertain digit. This means that the final recorded digit is considered to be uncertain. Every calculated value using collected data has uncertainty. Significant figures determine where to round when doing calculations with data. Also, significant figures prevent the answers to calculations from being stated with higher precision than the data used in the calculation would actually support.

When using significant figures in calculations, there are two sets of rules: one for addition and subtraction, and one for multiplication and division. For addition and subtraction calculations, answers should be rounded to the leftmost uncertain digit. For example, when adding measurements of 2.3 g and 10.81 g, the correct answer would be 13.1 g. The first term's uncertain digit is in the tenths place, while the second term's uncertain digit is in the hundredths place. Thus, the answer is rounded to the tenths place. In multiplication and division calculations, answers should be rounded to the exact number of significant figures in the factor that has the smallest number of significant figures. For example, when multiplying 3.2 by 4.001, the correct answer may only have 2 significant figures because 3.2 only has 2 significant figures. Therefore, the correct answer is 13. If the first factor were instead 3.20 or 3.200 (indicating that this value was known with greater precision), the answer would be 12.8 or 12.80, respectively.

DATA ERRORS AND ERROR ANALYSIS

No measurements are ever 100% accurate. There is always some amount of error regardless of how careful the observer or how good his equipment. The important thing for the scientist to know is how much error is present in a given measurement. Two commonly misunderstood terms regarding error are accuracy and precision. Accuracy is a measure of how close a measurement is to the true value. Precision is a measure of how close repeated measurements are to one another. Error is usually quantified using a confidence interval and an uncertainty value. For instance, if the quantity is measured as 100 ± 2 on a 95% confidence interval, this means that there is a 95% chance that the actual value falls between 98 and 102.

DATA ANALYSIS

The **measure of central tendency** is a statistical value that gives a general tendency for the center of a group of data. There are several different ways of describing the measure of central tendency. Each one has a unique way it is calculated, and each one gives a slightly different perspective on the data set. Whenever you give a measure of central tendency, always make sure the units are the same. If the data has different units, such as hours, minutes, and seconds, convert all the data to the same unit, and use the same unit in the measure of central tendency. If no units are given in the data, do not give units for the measure of central tendency.

MEAN

The statistical **mean** of a group of data is the same as the arithmetic average of that group. To find the mean of a set of data, first convert each value to the same units, if necessary. Then find the sum of all the values, and count the total number of data values, making sure you take into consideration each individual value. If a value appears more than once, count it more than once. Divide the sum of the values by the total number of values and apply the units, if any. Note that the mean does not have to be one of the data values in the set, and may not divide evenly.

$$\text{mean} = \frac{\text{sum of the data values}}{\text{quantity of data values}}$$

While the mean is relatively easy to calculate and averages are understood by most people, the mean can be very misleading if it is used as the sole measure of central tendency. If the data set has outliers (data values that are unusually high or unusually low compared to the rest of the data values), the mean can be very distorted, especially if the data set has a small number of values. If unusually high values are countered with unusually low values, the mean is not affected as much. For example, if five of twenty students in a class get a 100 on a test, but the other 15 students have an average of 60 on the same test, the class average would appear as 70. Whenever the mean is skewed by outliers, it is always a good idea to include the median as an alternate measure of central tendency.

MEDIAN

The statistical **median** is the value in the middle of the set of data. To find the median, list all data values in order from smallest to largest or from largest to smallest. Any value that is repeated in the set must be listed the number of times it appears. If there are an odd number of data values, the median is the value in the middle of the list. If there is an even number of data values, the median is the arithmetic mean of the two middle values.

The big disadvantage of using the median as a measure of central tendency is that is relies solely on a value's relative size as compared to the other values in the set. When the individual values in a set of data are evenly dispersed, the median can be an accurate tool. However, if there is a group of rather large values or a group of rather small values that are not offset by a different group of values, the information that can be inferred from the median may not be accurate because the distribution of values is skewed.

MODE

The statistical **mode** is the data value that occurs the most frequently in the data set. It is possible to have exactly one mode, more than one mode, or no mode. To find the mode of a set of data, arrange the data like you do to find the median (all values in order, listing all multiples of data values). Count the number of times each value appears in the data set. If all values appear an equal number of times, there is no mode. If one value appears more than any other value, that value is the mode. If two or more values appear the same number of times, but there are other values that appear fewer times and no values that appear more times, all of those values are the modes.

The main disadvantage of the mode is that the values of the other data in the set have no bearing on the mode. The mode may be the largest value, the smallest value, or a value anywhere in between in the set. The mode only tells which value or values, if any, occurred the greatest number of times. It does not give any suggestions about the remaining values in the set.

BEER'S LAW

Beer's law is defined as $A = abc$, where A is the absorbance, a is the absorptivity, b is the path of light in centimeters (cm), and c is the concentration of the absorbing compound. Consider the following example:

For a certain spectrophotometric procedure, the absorbance of a standard solution (concentration is 25 mg/dL) is 0.75 (in a 1 cm cell). The absorbance of the sample solution is 0.35 (in a 1 cm cell). Calculate the concentration of the sample solution.

Both b (the path of light in centimeters) and a (the absorptivity) are constant. So, using Beer's law, the equation for the relationship is: $\frac{c_{sample}}{c_{standard}} = \frac{A_{sample}}{A_{standard}}$. All of the values in that equation are known except for the concentration of the sample:

$$c_{sample} = \frac{A_{sample} \times c_{standard}}{A_{standard}}$$
$$= \frac{0.35 \times 25}{0.75} \frac{mg}{dL}$$
$$= 11.7 \text{ mg/dL}$$

MOLARITY AND MOLALITY OF A SOLUTION

Molarity and molality are measures of the concentration of a solution. Molarity (M) is the amount of solute in moles per the amount of solution in liters. A 1.0 M solution consists of 1.0 mole of solute for each 1.0 L of solution. Molality (m) is the amount of solute in moles per the amount of solvent in kilograms. A 1.0 m solution consists of 1.0 mole of solute for each 1.0 kg of solvent. Often, when performing these calculations, the amount of solute is given in grams. To convert from grams of solute to moles of solute, multiply the grams of solute by the molar mass of the solute:

$$Molarity\ (M) = \frac{moles\ of\ solute\ (mol)}{liters\ of\ solution\ (L)}$$

$$Molality\ (m) = \frac{moles\ of\ solute\ (mol)}{kilograms\ of\ solvent\ (kg)}$$

MOLARITY OF A SOLUTION EXAMPLE

Determine the molarity of a solution that contains 20.0 grams of NaCl in 500 mL of solution.

The molarity of a solution is equal to moles per liter. In this example, we need to calculate what one mole (gram molecular weight) is of NaCl first. A mole of a compound is equal to the sum of the atomic weights of the elements in that compound. So, for NaCl, one mole is equal to the atomic weight of sodium plus the atomic weight of chlorine, $23.0\frac{g}{mol} + 35.5\frac{g}{mol} = 58.5\frac{g}{mol}$. Next, it is best to determine the concentration of the solution in terms of grams per liter. So, in our example, the solution is $\frac{20.0\ g}{500\ mL}$. This is equivalent to $\frac{20.0\ g}{0.5\ L} = 40\frac{g}{L}$. Next, the number of moles of NaCl present in the solution must be calculated. Take the grams of NaCl present in 1 liter of solution and divide it by the weight of one mole of NaCl: $\frac{40\ g}{58.5\frac{g}{mol}} = 0.68$ mol. Since molarity is equal to moles per liter, the molarity of this solution is therefore $0.68\frac{mol}{L}$, or the solution is a 0.68 M NaCl solution.

OSMOLALITY

Osmolality is defined as the moles per 1 kilogram (kg) of solvent multiplied by the number of particles into which the molecules of solute dissociate. For instance, consider calculating the osmolality of 54 g glucose and 11.7 g NaCl in 2 kg of water.

To calculate the osmolality, first we need to calculate how many moles of solute (both glucose and NaCl) are present.

For glucose, $54\ g = \frac{54\ g}{180\frac{g}{mol}} = 0.3$ mol. For NaCl, $11.7\ g = \frac{11.7\ g}{58.5\frac{g}{mol}} = 0.2$ mol.

Then, we need to look at how each solute dissociates. Glucose does not dissociate. However, 0.2 mol NaCl will dissociate into two particles, 0.2 mol Na^+ and 0.2 mol Cl^-. So, to calculate the number of osmoles (Osm) present, we would add 0.3 Osm glucose to 0.2 Osm Na^+ and 0.2 Osm Cl^-. This totals 0.7 Osm present. Because we are dealing with 2 kg of water, however, and osmolality is noted as moles per kilogram, we need to divide 0.7 Osm by 2 kg of water, to give an osmolality of 0.35.

PREPARING A SOLUTION EXAMPLE

Determine how many grams of KCl are required to prepare 250 mL of a 3 M solution.

A 1 M solution is equal to 1 mole of solute divided by 1 liter of solution. To begin, the molecular weight of 1 mole of KCl must be calculated: $39.1 \text{ g} + 35.5 \text{ g} = 74.6 \text{ g}$. Therefore, 1 liter of a 1 M solution of KCl contains 74.6 g. However, since we are interested in a 3 M solution, the number of grams contained in a 1 M solution must be multiplied by 3. Therefore, a 3 M solution contains $3 \times 74.6 \frac{g}{L} = 223.8 \frac{g}{L}$. In this case, though, only 250 mL or 0.250 L of the 3 M solution are needed. So, the 3 M solution needs to be multiplied by the volume needed. This equation then becomes: $223.8 \frac{g}{L} \times 0.250 \text{ L} = 56.0 \text{ g KCl}$. Therefore, in order to prepare 250 mL of a 3 M solution of KCl, 56.0 g of KCl are needed.

PREPARING A DILUTE SOLUTION FROM A STOCK SOLUTION

In order to prepare a dilute solution from a stock solution, the molarity and the needed volume of the diluted solution as well as the molarity of the stock solution must be known. The volume of the stock solution to be diluted can be calculated using the formula $V_{stock}M_{stock} = V_{dilute}M_{dilute}$, where V_{stock} is the unknown variable, M_{stock} is the molarity of the stock solution, V_{dilute} is the needed volume of the dilute solution, and M_{dilute} is the needed molarity of the dilute solution. Solving this formula for V_{stock} yields $V_{stock} = \frac{V_{dilute}M_{dilute}}{M_{stock}}$. Then, dilute the calculated amount of stock solution (V_{stock}) to the total volume required of the diluted solution.

DETERMINING FINAL CONCENTRATIONS OF SOLUTIONS EXAMPLES

When calculating a final concentration of a solution after multiple dilutions, the initial concentration of the solution is multiplied by each of the dilutions as a fraction. Consider the following examples:

A 2 M solution diluted 2:5 and then diluted 1:4

To calculate the final concentration of this 2 M solution after being diluted 2:5 and 1:4, the equation used would be $(2 \text{ M}) \times \frac{2}{5} \times \frac{1}{4}$. The final concentration would then be 0.2 M.

A 5 M solution diluted 1:2, then diluted 2:3, and then diluted 3:5

In this situation, the equation used to calculate the final concentration of the solution after undergoing multiple dilutions as stated would be $(5 \text{ M}) \times \frac{1}{2} \times \frac{2}{3} \times \frac{3}{5}$. The final concentration of this solution is then calculated to be 1 M.

A 4 M solution diluted 3:7, then diluted 6:13, and then diluted 1:2

In this particular situation, the equation used to calculate the final concentration of the solution after undergoing three separate dilutions as stated in the problem would be $(4 \text{ M}) \times \frac{3}{7} \times \frac{6}{13} \times \frac{1}{2}$. Using this equation, the final concentration of the solution can be calculated to be approximately 0.4 M.

CALCULATING CONCENTRATION IN MILLIEQUIVALENTS PER LITER

To calculate a concentration in milliequivalents per liter when given concentration in milligrams per deciliter, the following equation needs to be used:

$$\frac{\frac{mg}{dL} \times \frac{10\ dL}{L} \times valence}{atomic\ mass} = mEq/L$$

Calculate the concentration in milliequivalents per liter ($\frac{mEq}{L}$) of a serum potassium level of 22.3 $\frac{mg}{dL}$.

For potassium, the valence is 1, and the atomic mass is 39. These values can be obtained by using a periodic table. Therefore, the equation then becomes:

$$\frac{\left(22.3\ \frac{mg}{dL}\right) \times \left(\frac{10\ dL}{L}\right) \times 1}{39\ \frac{g}{mol}} = 5.7\ mEq/L$$

Calculate the concentration in milliequivalents per liter of a serum calcium level of 9.0 $\frac{mg}{dL}$.

For calcium, the valence is 2, and the atomic mass is 40. Therefore:

$$\frac{\left(9.0\ \frac{mg}{dL}\right) \times \left(\frac{10\ dL}{L}\right) \times 2}{40\ \frac{g}{mol}} = 4.5\ mEq/L$$

SENSITIVITY, SPECIFICITY, AND PREDICTIVE VALUE

Getting answers with a high probability of being accurate is the best that can be hoped for in a medical test. A test can produce two kinds of errors: a false positive result (meaning that the presence of disease is detected when there is, in fact, no disease) or a false negative result indicating no disease is present when it actually is.

- Test **sensitivity**: Measures a screening test's ability to correctly identify the presence of a disease, it is the ratio of tests with positive outcomes to the total number of affected (true positive) patients tested.
- Test **specificity**: Measures a screening test's ability to correctly identify the absence of disease.

A test with both high sensitivity and high specificity can be expected to have high **predictive value**.

- True-positive (TP): the test is positive, and the patient has acquired a disease.
- False-positive (FP): the test is positive but the patient does not have the disease.
- True-negative (TN): the test is negative, but the patient does not have a disease.
- False-negative (FN): the test is negative; the patient does have the disease.
- Level of sensitivity in testing: probability of a positive test result when a patient has the disease, as indicated by the ratio, TP/(TP + FN).
- Degree of specificity: the probability that a negative test truly indicates a disease-free patient, represented by the ratio, TN/(TN + FP).

- Positive predictive value: the probability that a test will produce positive results for patients who have the disease, indicated in the ratio, TP/(TP + FP).
- Negative predictive value: denotes the probability that no disease exists in patients testing negative, stated in the ratio: TN/(TN + FN).

Manual and Automated Methodology and Instrumentation

SETTING UP, BALANCING, AND OPERATING A CENTRIFUGE

Centrifuges spin solutions to separate out solid materials by forcing them away from the center to form a pellet. Centrifuges come in various sizes and may be free floating/horizontal or angle-head (45-degree angle). Different specimens require different G-forces or **relative centrifugal force** (RCF) and different durations. The RCF is the spinning force relative to Earth's gravitation and depends on the revolutions per minute (RPM) and the radius of revolution (RR) measured in mm from the center to the end of the test tube (It can also be found using a nomogram chart.):

$$RCF = 1.12 \times RR \times \left(\frac{RPM}{1000}\right)^2$$

Procedure:

1. Use equal numbers of tubes in the buckets on opposite sites. Weigh tubes to ensure the load is balanced and use a tube filled with water if testing an odd number.
2. Close and lock centrifuge, turn it on, and follow instructions for settings.
3. Spin for necessary duration (such as 15 to 20 minutes). If excessive vibration (from imbalance) or sound of cracking vial occurs, turn off machine.
4. When completed, remove buckets carefully to avoid jarring the pellets.
5. Open buckets and remove tubes, checking for sediments.

MICROSCOPES

The microscope most commonly used is the **light microscope** (either monocular or binocular). This microscope uses external light or light from an internal filament that allows the light to pass upward through the specimen so that the specimen appears dark against the lighter background, although the light may be inverted, illuminating from the top, for such things as a culture in a liquid medium. **Phase contrast microscopes** that do not require staining of the specimen are used to assess cell growth, especially for organisms that are transparent with standard light microscope. The **dark field microscope** uses a special dark-field condenser that makes the specimen appear light against a dark background, useful for observing spirochetes. The **fluorescent microscope** utilizes an ultraviolet light for illumination. This microscope is used when fluorescent dye is attached to a specimen because the dye glows when exposed to ultraviolet light, useful for fluorescent antibody testing.

OCULAR MICROMETER

The ocular micrometer is a glass disk that fits into the microscope eyepiece and provides an engraved ruler for measurement within the ocular lens. The **ocular micrometer calibration** procedure is as follows:

1. Remove eyepiece and unscrew the ocular eye lens and position the ocular micrometer with the engraved ruler with 100 divisions face down, replace the lens, and place the ocular with the micrometer into the ocular tube and microscope with 10× objective.
2. Place a stage micrometer slide with an engraved scale that closely matches in the ocular micrometer length and number of divisions on the microscope stage and focus on the parallel sets of rulers so that the 0-mm lines on the ocular micrometer and stage micrometer align.
3. Locate another set of lines that align at the furthest distance from the 0-mm lines.
4. Count the number of lines between the 0-mm alignment and the distant alignment on both the ocular micrometer scale and the stage micrometer scale.
5. Use formulas to determine the proportion of a mm measured by 1 ocular unit:
6. Stage micrometer reading × 1000 micrometers/ocular micrometer reading × 1 mm = ocular units.
7. For 40× objective: 0.1 mm × 1000 micrometer/50 units × 1 mm.

MANUAL INSTRUMENTATION

Borosilicate glassware is heat and chemical resistant; soda lime glassware, less expensive and less resistant; and plastic ware, less expensive and less breakable but not heat resistant and cannot be used with some reagents and chemicals. Commonly used manual laboratory instrumentation includes:

- **Test tubes**: Used to heat and hold reagents to assess chemical reactions. Vary in size and usually rimless. Held in plastic or metal test tube racks. Centrifuge tubes (15 mL) are similar but have tapered ends to hold pellet. Cuvettes are rectangular test tubes to hold solutions for photometry, placed only in plastic racks to avoid scratching.
- **Funnels (plain and separating)**: Supported in ring stand and used for filtration or to separate immiscible liquids.
- **General purpose and volumetric glassware**: Includes graduated cylinders, volumetric flasks, pipettes, and burettes and used for measuring volumes. Pipettes or eyedroppers are used to transfer liquids. Mouth pipettes should never be used. Reagent bottles hold reagents. Beakers are used to heat liquids.

Cleaning and maintenance of manual instrumentation: All glassware and plastic ware should be rinsed immediately after use in hot tap water to prevent substances from drying. The rinsed ware is soaked in low suds detergent solution (2%) for at least an hour. The ware is then scrubbed with appropriately-sized brushes inside and out. Chromic acid may be used to remove coagulated organic material. Each item is washed 5 times under running tap water to remove all detergent followed by 3 rinses with distilled or deionized water. After the washing and rinsing are completed, the equipment is dried in an oven at 140 °C if heat resistant or placed in a drying rack overnight. Prior to first use of newly purchased glassware, items made of borosilicate glass should be cleaned with detergent, washed under tap water, and rinsed with distilled/deionized water. Items made of soda lime glass should be soaked overnight in 5% hydrochloric acid, diluted 6 times to 30% to neutralize free alkali before washing under tap water, and rinsed with distilled/deionized water.

ADVANTAGES AND DISADVANTAGES OF AUTOMATED LABORATORY INSTRUMENTATION

Automated laboratory instrumentation is becoming the norm, and a laboratory may have total laboratory automation or system-based automation. Automated laboratory instrumentation has a number of advantages over manual procedures:

- Test results can be obtained faster and are often more accurate because they are not dependent on varying techniques and subjective judgment.
- Test results are more reliable and consistent, and can be easily reproduced.
- Data can be more easily stored, transferred, manipulated, and reported.
- Fewer laboratory personnel are needed because the automated systems can do the work of many technicians.
- Errors are minimized.
- Workflow is more efficient.

However, there are also some disadvantages: If a machine breaks down, there may be considerable delay in manually producing lab reports because of inadequate staffing or equipment. Additionally, staff members must be trained in trouble shooting and maintenance of equipment and service technicians must be available. The automation equipment may be prohibitively expensive, especially for a small laboratory.

MASS SPECTROMETRY

Mass spectrometry (MS) analysis allows for the separation, detection, and measurement of individual sample components by their mass and electrical charge. MS achieves the ionization of a solid, liquid, or gaseous sample by various methods, breaking large molecules into charged fragments or pulling electrons off of small molecules or atoms. Ionized products are moved to the next phase of analysis where they are focused into a beam and accelerated to increase kinetic energy. The ion beam then passes through a magnetic field, and the ions are deflected at different speeds and angles, with some hitting the detector. The detection of various separated ions can be completed in a single run by careful tuning of the magnetic field, flow rate of the sample, energy applied to the ionization, and other key properties. Data produced by the mass spectrometer are plotted by the mass-to-charge ratio of components present in a sample and compared to known results of various compounds.

MS is highly sensitive and has the capability to produce qualitative and quantitative results. Although MS can be a stand-alone process, it is most often used in conjunction with chromatography techniques for clear and reliable results. Automation of the process from preanalytical to postanalytical allows for a more efficient workflow for laboratory staff because the analytical process is meticulous and time-consuming.

CHROMATOGRAPHY

Chromatography methodologies are used in the laboratory to separate one particular component in a mixture. Chromatography requires two phases: a mobile phase and a fixed or stationary phase. The **mobile phase** is a mixture of solutes dissolved into a reagent that moves through the stationary phase. The **stationary phase** consists of specifically chosen and prepared compounds that are adhered to a column, tube, or sheet. As the mobile phase passes through the stationary phase, the solutes in the mobile phase interact with the compounds of the stationary phase and get slowed down. However, different solutes are slowed to varying degrees and, as such, the constituents of the mobile phase get separated.

Chromatography can be done with either gas or liquid. Gas chromatography methodologies require a columnar capillary tube as the stationary phase, whereas liquid chromatography can use various fixed structures. Flat structures used for the stationary phase include sheets of cellulose paper or a thin layer of glass or plastic. Liquid chromatography can also be performed with a columnar stationary phase similar to a capillary tube. This method is what is most often used in conjunction with mass spectrometry. Due to the increased precision, higher speeds of separation, and increasing complexity of samples, chromatography has shifted from a manual method to being performed by automated instrumentation.

Basic Management Principles

STAFFING AND FUNCTIONS

Laboratory staffing structures are based on a combination of the professional and educational experience of its members. An appropriately structured staff determines the supervision, decision, and resolution responsibilities belonging to each staff member. The **medical director** of a lab typically must have a PhD in pathology, an MD, or a DO degree. Pathologists in the position of medical director may specialize in anatomic pathology, clinical pathology, or both. The medical director is responsible for the laboratory's scope, standard of service, and quality of service with regard to the legal, moral, and ethical aspects. **Laboratory managers** are most often a certified medical laboratory scientist (MLS) with an advanced degree and administrative experience. Managers are responsible for the technical, administrative, and legal aspects of a laboratory, including compliance of legal operating conditions and balanced, cost-effective work performance. Clear and concise communication to laboratory staff and to others who use laboratory services is crucial for successful laboratory management. **Laboratory supervisors** are MLSs that manage the technical aspects of the laboratory including quality control, analytes, and instrument maintenance. **Technologists** and **technicians** perform clinical assays as well as teach, train, and supervise support staff members. Technologists have completed a four-year college degree, whereas technicians hold a two-year degree. Various positions within the laboratory are considered as **support staff.** Responsibilities of the support staff include clerical, specimen processing, laboratory assisting, and phlebotomy.

MEDICAL/PROFESSIONAL ETHICS

In general, **ethics** is defined as a set of principles that help navigate dealing with the good and the bad. **Personal** codes of ethics are specific to each individual, **professional** codes of ethics are principles determined for the appropriate conduct of an individual or group in the workplace, and **medical** codes of ethics are principles specific to conduct and problem resolution in a clinical setting. Each decision that laboratory professionals make requires the application of personal, professional, and medical ethics in order to properly care for patients while supporting themselves, their coworkers, and the organization they represent.

The American Society for Clinical Laboratory Science (ASCLS) has published a professional code of ethics specific to laboratory personnel. The code expresses that all laboratory professionals have the responsibility of practicing proper conduct toward their patients, their colleagues, the profession, and society as a whole. The ASCLS code of ethics outlines laboratory professionals' duty to the following populations and their purpose:

- **Duty to patients**: Laboratory professionals' primary duty is to maintain the welfare of patients by providing the highest quality of care by accounting for the quality and integrity of laboratory services, practicing within their limits, and respecting patient privacy and confidentiality.

- **Duty to colleagues:** Act in a manner that promotes the dignity and respect of the profession and establishes a respectful work environment. Uphold the standards of the profession through competency, honesty, integrity, and reliability.
- **Duty to society:** Contribute to the general well-being of society by striving to improve patient outcomes and serving as patient advocates.

MEDICAL LEGAL INFORMATION

There are several legal terms that laboratory professionals must familiarize themselves with because some are a part of the laboratory's day-to-day functions. Prior to the performance of laboratory-related procedures, consent must be obtained from a patient in one of the following ways:

Implied consent describes the assumption of a patient's agreement to simple, routine procedures simply by their entrance to a healthcare facility. Venipuncture is a laboratory procedure that falls under the category of implied consent.

Informed consent is defined as a patient's full awareness and understanding of a test or procedure being completed. Informed consent is required for more complex procedures, and it requires the patient to be fully informed of the process and how their results will be managed following the procedure. In cases regarding minors and legally incompetent adults, their legal guardians must be informed and must sign any consent forms on their behalf. Bone marrow aspirates, spinal taps, fine needle aspirations, and blood transfusions are laboratory-based procedures that require informed consent by a patient.

STANDARD OF CARE AND CHAIN OF CUSTODY

The well-being and safety of patients must be the top priority for all healthcare professionals. In efforts to protect and support patients from unnecessary harm, a standard of care has been created. The **standard of care** represents the appropriate degree of care that a reasonable healthcare professional would take to prevent injury or harm to a patient or another person. Failure to follow the standard of care that results in an injury or death may be considered medical negligence. Individuals negatively affected by the event have the right to sue for damages.

The **chain of custody** is a documentation process that must be followed for records and laboratory findings to be considered admissible in court. The collection, transport, analysis, and results of lab samples must be thoroughly documented with the dates, times, and initials of staff for the chain of custody to remain intact. The purpose of the chain of custody is to establish the certainty that a specimen was not altered in any way that would change its admissibility. Laboratory sample results that may be used in court include the following: blood or breath alcohol levels, specimens obtained from victims of sexual abuse, paternity tests, and specimens from a medical examiner. Although every sample will not be used in a court case, laboratories follow chain of custody documentation guidelines for all specimens. This allows for consistency in documentation and effective specimen tracking, and it ensures that chain of custody requirements are met in the event a sample is required in a court of law.

HEALTH INSURANCE PORTABILITY AND ACCOUNTABILITY ACT

The Health Insurance Portability and Accountability Act of 1996 (**HIPAA**) provides a set of rules and regulations for healthcare professionals and facilities to follow regarding the confidentiality of patient's protected health information (**PHI**). HIPAA states that patients have a right to know and approve of who has access to their private healthcare information. Information covered under HIPAA includes any identifiable detail or demographic linked to an individual's physical or mental health and records regarding payment of healthcare. Typically, laboratory staff have access to the majority or all of a patient's protected information via the integration of electronic health records and hospital information systems with laboratory information systems. HIPAA allows for laboratory professionals to access PHI only when it is pertinent to their job function and it is required for the completion of a job-related task.

Under HIPAA, the following instances are examples of appropriate laboratory staff use of PHI:

- Patient demographics and insurance information for registration purposes
- Patient demographics and reportable disease laboratory results to provide to public health departments
- Previous diagnosis and laboratory reports for verification, correlation, or troubleshooting current laboratory results
- Patient results and demographics for ordering providers when communicating a critical laboratory value

The following instances are examples of inappropriate laboratory staff use of PHI:

- Accessing laboratory results or other healthcare information on oneself, friends, family members, patients, or others without permission or when it is not necessary for a job-related task
- Sharing patient demographics or health records with others without patient consent or when it is not necessary for a specific job-related task
- Openly speaking of patients' health information in an identifiable manner without their consent

Education Principles

LABORATORY INFORMATION MANAGEMENT SYSTEMS AND AUTOMATION

A **laboratory information management system** (LIMS) is a specimen-based system that is used to integrate automation and uniform methodologies to the laboratory in order to increase productivity, data management, and process integrity. Although a LIMS can be tailored to each laboratory's specific needs, it must also meet the following requirements: secure logins, flexibility for software updates and add-ons, and the ability to manage data. In addition to LIMS, laboratories are becoming further automated by integration with the laboratory information system (LIS). The **LIS** is a patient-based system that provides clinical information including patient demographics, diagnosis, and laboratory results, in one place. Integration of LIMS and LIS into laboratory processes allows for increased productivity, decreased risk of data and clerical errors, and the direct delivery of patients' results to providers for review, medical records, and billing purposes. Automation supports an accurate and efficient workflow for laboratory professionals and allows for more precision in patient care. Laboratory automation achieves these goals in the following ways:

- Built-in tools and accessibility promote compliance with regulations and standard operating procedures.
- Analyzer interfaces receive results directly from instrumentation and point-of-care equipment.
- Rule-based logic and calculations are formulated and automatically applied when necessary.

- Quality control functionality and data storage are organized for efficient review and management.
- Data entry, result interpretation, and report generation and distribution are more accurate and efficient.

LIS APPLICATIONS

The **LIS** electronically manages patient and laboratory data throughout each stage of the analytical process, increasing work efficiency and decreasing the risk of error. In multispecialty facilities, hospital information system networks and LIS are linked together for patient information to be easily viewed and accessed in both programs. The **preanalytical** process begins with patient registration. Upon first admission to the hospital information system, patients receive a medical record number, with each new admission generating a unique account number linked to all services for a specific visit. Patient medical record numbers and account numbers provide pertinent patient demographics to the LIS. Laboratory test orders entered into the LIS automatically generate requisitions and specimen bar codes, providing detailed electronic documentation of specimen collection, tracking, and processing. LIS automation of the **analytical** phase allows laboratory analyzers to link sample bar codes to LIS test requisitions and perform the appropriate tests on each sample. Following sample analysis, analyzers transfer test results directly into the LIS for manual review and **postanalytical** verification by lab staff. Autoverification of normal test results can be completed by the LIS using mathematical algorithms based on laboratory policies. This process automatically reviews and verifies results without the need for manual review by staff, increasing productivity and time management. Finally, reports of laboratory results are generated by the LIS and can be electronically transmitted to printers, computers, and pagers for remote and rapid access to results.

COMPETENCY TESTING AND PROFICIENCY SURVEYS

Competency testing is a method of evaluating an individual's ability to meet job-specific requirements using their knowledge, skills, and experience. Laboratories are required to evaluate employees for competency upon hiring, after 60 days of employment, and annually thereafter. Assessing the competence of laboratory staff ensures that they are fulfilling their job duties and properly following rules and regulations, while also detecting deficiencies and allowing for quality and process improvements to be made.

Participation in **proficiency surveys** is required by laboratory accrediting associations to monitor and improve the quality of routine analytics performed by a laboratory. Samples with unknown concentrations are provided to laboratories for each analyte or procedure that is routinely performed in the facility. Proficiency samples are to be tested following the same procedures and using the same equipment as patient samples, and the obtained results are reported back to the company providing the samples. Several laboratories receive the same samples, which allows for interlaboratory comparison of results obtained from different facilities. The objective of proficiency testing is to provide evidence of a competent lab staff, proficient standard operating procedures, and properly functioning instrumentation.

MLS Practice Test

1. Receiving cannot accept a specimen unless it has:

    a.   A correct, legible label
    b.   An uncontaminated, signed requisition with billing information
    c.   An intact container with correct media
    d.   All of the above

2. A laboratory refrigerator used to store volatile, flammable liquids can hold:

    a.   120 gallons of class I, II, and IIIA liquids
    b.   180 gallons of class I, II, and IIIA liquids
    c.   200 gallons of class I, II, and IIIA liquids
    d.   50 gallons of class I, II, and IIIA liquids

3. Disease incidence predicts:

    a.   How probable it is a patient will develop a disease, and its etiology
    b.   How likely a test result is to be right or wrong, given certain variables
    c.   How likely the patient with a negative test really does not have the condition
    d.   How likely the patient with a positive test result really has the condition

4. Beer's law in spectrophotometry

    a.   Means a transparent sample transmits 0% light
    b.   Only applies if absorbance is between 0.1 and 1.0
    c.   Means an opaque sample transmits 100% light
    d.   Uses a visible spectrum from 340 nm to 500 nm

5. Naming bacteria by looking at their size and shape under the microscope, and the colony morphology on media is:

    a.   Differential identification
    b.   Numeric taxonomy
    c.   Presumptive identification
    d.   *TaqMan* electrophoresis

6. OSHA allows ungloved phlebotomy only if:

    a.   The experienced phlebotomist working in a volunteer blood donor center agrees.
    b.   The phlebotomist's skin is intact and the patient is cooperative.
    c.   Both a and b
    d.   The patient is an infant.

7. The hospital department that studies alcohol, drugs, poisons, and heavy metals is:

    a.   Serology/Immunology
    b.   Toxicology
    c.   Cytology
    d.   Endocrinology

8. A hemoglobin electrophoresis result of adult hemoglobin (HbA) or HbA$_2$ means the patient has:

    a. Sickle cell anemia

    b. Fetal hemoglobin

    c. Normal hemoglobin

    d. Hemolytic anemia

9. US law overrides the patient's right to confidentiality if:

    a. The patient has a sexually transmitted disease or tuberculosis (TB)

    b. The caregiver is likely to be infected

    c. Authorities suspect child abuse or neglect under CAPTA

    d. All of the above

10. The recall rate is also known as the:

    a. Sensitivity

    b. Specificity

    c. Aliquot

    d. Circadian rhythm

11. Biochemistry usually requires:

    a. Lavender, light blue, and black blood collection tubes

    b. Red, pink, and yellow blood collection tubes

    c. Green, gray, and marbled serum-separator tube (SST) blood collection tubes

    d. Navy, purple, and brown blood collection tubes

12. A normal kidney function study shows a:

    a. BUN to creatinine ratio between 15:1 and 20:1

    b. Alkaline phosphatase 30–85 international milliunits/mL

    c. Serum aspartate aminotransferase 5–40 international units/L

    d. Amylase 56–190 international units/L

13. A newborn's jaundice could be caused by:

    a. Erythroblastosis fetalis

    b. Kernicterus

    c. Physiologic jaundice from poor fluid intake

    d. All of the above

14. Lipids from carbohydrate and alcohol sources are:

    a. Anions

    b. Triglycerides

    c. Cholesterol

    d. Eluent

15. When serum proteins indicates disease, the doctor usually follows up with:

    a. Total protein, albumin, and globulin

    b. Ascites

    c. Protein electrophoresis

    d. Bilirubin

16. Elevated creatine phosphokinase (CPK) could mean myocardial infarction, but could also mean:

a. Alcoholism, hypothyroidism, cardioversion, or clofibrate use
b. Aspirin, burns, warfarin, or sickle cell anemia
c. Lung disease or congestive heart failure
d. Crushing injury, bowel infarction, or opiate use

17. A patient whose cortisol level is high at both 8:00 a.m. and 4:00 p.m. likely has:

a. Addison's disease
b. Natriuretic factor
c. Diabetes insipidus
d. Cushing syndrome

18. Decreased sodium in the blood is:

a. Hypernatremia, often from diabetes, burns, or Cushing syndrome
b. Hyponatremia, often from vomiting and diarrhea, furosemide, or Addison's disease
c. Hyperkalemia, often from acidosis, spironolactone, or kidney failure
d. Hypokalemia, often from alkalosis, stomach cancer, or eating too much licorice

19. CPK in a patient with a myocardial infarction will:

a. Rise 6 hours after heart attack, peak in 18 hours, and return to baseline in 3 days
b. Rise 6–10 hours after heart attack, peak at 12–48 hours, and return to baseline in 4 days
c. Rise 24–72 hours after heart attack, peak in 4 days, and return to baseline in 14 days
d. Cause a corresponding rise in alpha-fetoprotein

20. The panic value for blood pH is:

a. 7.35
b. Less than 7.20
c. 80–100 torr
d. 4.0–8.0 mcg/L

21. The liver destroys old blood cells at the end of their lifespan of:

a. 120 days
b. 30 days
c. 1 week
d. 90 days

22. An erythrocyte sedimentation rate (ESR) measures how blood cells with anticoagulant aggregate in a Westergren or Wintrobe tube in 1 hour because of changes in plasma proteins, which is known as :

a. Retic count
b. Serendipity
c. Fibrinolysis
d. Rouleaux formation

23. If the doctor suspects the patient has Hodgkin disease, then the correct stain for the smear is:

    a. Periodic acid-Schiff (PAS)
    b. Sudan black B (SBB)
    c. Leukocyte alkaline phosphatase (LAP)
    d. Lactophenol cotton blue (LPCB)

24. A battlement scan is preferable to a wedge scan for studying bone marrow because:

    a. Battlement technique distributes cells evenly across the slide
    b. Lymphocytes concentrate in the feather
    c. Wedge technique causes leukocytes to pool in different sections of the slide
    d. Both a and c

25. Most coagulation (clotting) disorders are due to:

    a. Phase I problems
    b. Factor VIII deficiency
    c. Fibrinolysis
    d. Factor III distress call from the injury site

26. If the patient's PT and PTT are longer than 70 seconds, then check if _____ caused a false result:

    a. Ferritin
    b. Lupus inhibitor antibody (LA)
    c. Platelet antibody
    d. Intrinsic factor

27. Confirm a fungal infection found through microscopy with a:

    a. Latex serology for cryptococcal antigen
    b. Fungal serology titer of more than 1:32 that increases x4 or more 3 weeks later
    c. Complement fixation for coccidiomycosis and histoplasmosis
    d. Immunodiffusion for blastomycosis.

28. Two modern flocculation tests that replace the older Venereal Disease Research Laboratory (VDRL) test for syphilis screening are:

    a. Plasmacrit test (PCT) and rapid plasma reagin (RPR) test
    b. Fluorescent treponemal antibody absorption (FTA-ABS) and enzyme-linked immunosorbent assay (ELISA)
    c. Treponemal-specific microhemagglutination (MHA-TP) and *T. pallidum* particle agglutination test (TP-PA)
    d. Captia Syphilis-G enzyme immunoassay (EIA) and cold agglutinins

29. To make a dilution of ½ or 1:2

    a. Dilute ½ ml of serum with 2 mL of saline
    b. Dilute 1 ml of serum with 2 mL of saline
    c. Test undiluted serum for antibody/antigen reaction against a control
    d. Dilute 1 mL of serum with 1 mL of saline

30. A Monospot test uses ingredients from:
   a. Guinea pig, cow, and horse
   b. Sheep, pig, and horse
   c. Dog, sheep, and rabbit
   d. Fish, cat, and ferret

31. A prozone phenomenon occurs when performing an antibody titer on a patient with:
   a. Epstein-Barr virus (EBV)
   b. Reynaud disease
   c. Both syphilis and HIV
   d. Immunoglobulin G (IgG) antibodies

32. An Rh- mother who is pregnant with the child of an Rh+ father needs Rh immunoglobulin (*RhoGAM*):
   a. Even if the pregnancy ends in miscarriage or abortion
   b. At 26–28 weeks of pregnancy and again within 72 hours after her delivery.
   c. During her labor
   d. Both a and b

33. If your patient has a mild transfusion reaction:
   a. Eosinophilia, hypocalcemia, leukopenia, and pancytopenia may occur
   b. Dyscrasia, leukocytosis, hypercalcemia, and leukemia may occur
   c. Anemia, hypokalemia, glycosuria, and pancytopenia may occur
   d. Hemolysis, hyperkalemia, hypoglycemia, and hemoglobinuria may occur

34. Type O blood has:
   a. B antigen and anti-A antibody
   b. A antigen and anti-B antibody
   c. No A or B antigens and both anti-A and anti-B antibodies
   d. Both A and B antigens and no anti-A or anti-B antibodies

35. Choose the top priority transfusion patient from the list below.
   a. Cardiac surgery patient who lost more than 1,200 mL of blood
   b. Trauma patient with a hemoglobin of 5 g/dL
   c. Pernicious anemia patient
   d. Hemophiliac boy at regular clinic visit

36. Reject a transfusion request when:
   a. Recipient blood specimen is hemolyzed
   b. The patient armband does not have a unique identifier
   c. Donor blood is lipemic, clotted, or contains foreign objects
   d. All of the above

37. To diagnose a urinary tract infection correctly, the microbiology lab requires a:
   a. Midstream urine collection (MSU)
   b. Witnessed urine collection
   c. 24-hour urine collection
   d. Random urine collection

38. When assisting the doctor with cerebrospinal fluid (CSF) collection, you need 4 tubes for:

    a. Cell count, glucose and protein, gram stain and culture, virology/mycology/cytology.

    b. Immunoelectrophoresis

    c. Fungus, oncology, and SMA-12

    d. Neutrophilia, lymphocytophilia, glutamine, and lactate dehydrogenase (LDH)

39. Fusobacteria cause:

    a. Botulism and *Listeria* infections

    b. Lyme disease and *Helicobacter pylori* stomach ulcers

    c. Pyorrhea and Lemierre syndrome

    d. Chlamydia genital infections and pneumonia

40. The type of media required to incubate a TB culture correctly is:

    a. Tinsdale

    b. Sheep blood agar

    c. Modified Wadowsky-Yee (MWY)

    d. Löwenstein-Jensen (LJ) egg

41. To find parasites under the microscope, set the magnification to:

    a. 40x

    b. 10x

    c. 1000x

    d. 400x

42. Identify the parasite that must be reported to Public Health authorities:

    a. Crypto (Cryptosporidium parvum)

    b. Hookworm (Ancylostoma duodenale)

    c. Tapeworm (Cestoda)

    d. Pinworm (Enterobius)

43. To identify motile trophozoites:

    a. Examine blood smears and blood antigens

    b. Perform a string test

    c. Use *Snap n' Stain* on sputum

    d. Wet mount fresh, liquid stool with LPCB stain

44. Public Health requires you to keep positive parasitology samples preserved for :

    a. The patient's lifetime

    b. One year

    c. Ten years

    d. One month

45. Shine a Wood's lamp over the patient's skin to help you collect:

    a. Malaria specimens

    b. Public Health specimens

    c. Toxicology specimens

    d. Mycology specimens

46. Identify the positive dipstick test that would indicate an *E. coli* infection:

   a. Leukocytes
   b. Protein
   c. Ketones
   d. Nitrites

47. A pregnancy test may be ordered for a man with:

   a. Testicular cancer
   b. Prostatitis
   c. Cryptorchidism
   d. Peyronie disease

48. Normal urinary output for a 24-hour urine test is:

   a. 4 quarts
   b. 150–500 mL
   c. 30 liters
   d. 750–2,000 mL

49. Urate crystals found during microscopic urinalysis indicate:

   a. Urea-splitting bacteria are present
   b. Poisoning
   c. Gout
   d. Hyperparathyroidism

50. Patients with polycystic kidney disease (PKD) often have:

   a. Cirrhosis and hepatitis
   b. Coronary artery bypass graft (CABG) and hypertension
   c. Hematuria and uroliths
   d. Melena and hematochezia

51. Leukoreduced and irradiated platelet products are available to prevent platelet refractoriness caused by an incompatibility and alloimmunization of what antigen group?

   a. Rh antigens
   b. ABO antigens
   c. Class I HLA
   d. Class II HLA

52. Lewis, P1, Sd[a], and Chido and Rodgers antibodies bind with antigen-rich reagent serum to reveal antibodies present in a patient sample that are otherwise masked in which special blood bank technique?

   a. Elution
   b. Neutralization and inhibition
   c. Inactivation
   d. Adsorption

53. During hemoglobin A1C analysis, what laboratory method qualitatively detects hemoglobin variants by forcing them through a gradient at high pressures?

    a. Flow cytometry
    b. Gas chromatography-mass spectrometry
    c. High-performance liquid chromatography
    d. Liquid chromatography-tandem mass spectrometry

54. A patient is exhibiting bruising, excess bleeding, and a decreased response to commercial clotting factor therapy. Laboratory testing shows above-normal prothrombin time (PT), activated partial thromboplastin time (aPTT), and fibrinogen degradation product results as well as increased monoclonal immunoglobulin antibodies. What is the cause of this patient's condition?

    a. Acquired coagulation inhibitors
    b. Factor V deficiency
    c. Natural coagulation inhibitors
    d. Factor X deficiency

55. Following prolonged PT and aPTT results and a normal thrombin time (TT), what laboratory assay is performed next to detect and identify coagulation factor inhibitors?

    a. Lupus anticoagulant assays
    b. von Willebrand factor assays
    c. Factor assays
    d. Mixing studies

56. The activity of which of the following coagulation factors can be evaluated by PT-based and Russell's viper venom (RVV)-based factor assays?

    a. VII
    b. VIII
    c. X
    d. II

57. A patient is experiencing abnormal bleeding and is suspected of having a coagulation disorder. Laboratory assays produce the following results:

    Normal or elevated PTT
    Normal PT and platelet count
    Decreased factor VIII activity
    Decreased platelet aggregation with ristocetin

What disorder is most likely the cause of the patient's bleeding?

    a. Hemophilia A
    b. von Willebrand disease
    c. Factor IX deficiency
    d. Disseminated intravascular coagulation (DIC)

58. Which of the following platelet aggregation study agonists is used to induce granule release and stimulate platelet adhesion?

    a. Collagen
    b. Thrombin
    c. Arachidonic acid
    d. Adenosine diphosphate

59. What point-of-care assay tests the entire coagulation process and platelet function by measuring the viscoelastic properties of blood clot formation?

   a. Electrochemical international normalized ratio assay
   b. Bleeding time
   c. Platelet function assay
   d. Thromboelastography

60. Two days after heparin therapy, a patient presents with a platelet count declining to 110×10^{12}/L. A serotonin release assay and platelet factor 4 testing are ordered to diagnose what hypercoagulable condition?

   a. Immune heparin-induced thrombocytopenia (HIT)
   b. Nonimmune HIT
   c. Lupus anticoagulant
   d. Protein S activity

61. A patient with HIT has a baseline result of 28 seconds prior to beginning argatroban. During therapy, the patient must retain a result that is 1.5–3.0 times that of the baseline. What coagulation assay is being performed to determine the efficacy of the direct thrombin inhibitor being administered?

   a. PT
   b. Thrombin time (TT)
   c. Factor Xa inhibition assay
   d. PTT

62. A patient who is not receiving heparin therapy or exhibiting symptoms of a clotting disorder presents with an unexpectedly prolonged PTT. What is likely the cause of this result?

   a. Intravenous line contamination
   b. Clotting disorder
   c. Heparin neutralization from a heparinized tube
   d. Nothing, this is an expected result

63. Six weeks following the resolution of a painless lesion on the genitals, an individual displays a red rash that has diffused across the entire body, fatigue, and swollen lymph nodes. What stage of a *Treponema pallidum* infection is the individual experiencing?

   a. Primary
   b. Secondary
   c. Latent
   d. Tertiary

64. A patient returns 56 hours after receiving an intracutaneous injection in the forearm. The induration observed was <5 mm, indicating a negative result. Which method of tuberculosis (TB) testing was performed on this patient?

   a. Purified protein derivative skin test
   b. Interferon gamma release assay
   c. QuantiFERON assay
   d. Enzyme-linked immunosorbent assay (ELISA)

65. Which of the following testing techniques detects and identifies several cytokines at one time by using colored latex beads labeled with cytokine-specific antibodies?

    a. ELISA
    b. Multiplex immunoassay
    c. Rolling cycle amplification
    d. Chemiluminescent

66. The following target amplification process is performed:

    1. Primer 1 binds to the target nucleotide.
    2. Reverse transcriptase initiates polymerization of the strand.
    3. Reverse transcriptase with RNase H activity degrades the original target strand.

What is the next step in the process that allows for the target RNA amplicon molecule to be amplified?

    a. DNA polymerase extends to the primer, creating an altered strand that becomes the target for amplification.
    b. DNA polymerase adds nucleotides to the 3' end of each primer.
    c. Taq polymerase adds complementary bases; ligase anneals the appropriate primer to the target DNA probe.
    d. Primer 2 binds to the new synthesized strand. Elongation and polymerization form the RNA amplicon, a completed double strand of DNA.

67. A laboratory assay amplifies the viral RNA of HIV in a patient sample via the following procedure:

    1. Primer 1 hybridizes to the target RNA sequence.
    2. Reverse transcriptase elongates the primer's RNA copies to create a DNA/RNA hybrid.
    3. RNase H hydrolyzes the RNA portion, leaving a single-stranded DNA molecule.
    4. Primer 2 anneals to the DNA.
    5. Reverse transcriptase elongates primer 2, creating an active promotor site for transcription to occur.
    6. RNA polymerase produces multiple copies of RNA transcripts that are antisense to the original target sequence.

How is the concentration of viral RNA measured using this nucleic acid sequence-based amplification method?

    a. The molecular pattern produced that is plotted on a line graph
    b. Distance of migration of bands of genetic material
    c. Fluorescence emitted by target sequence and molecular beacon hybridization
    d. Based on the time elapsed before molecules elute off the capillary column

68. Under an ultraviolet fluorescent microscope, _____ are the portions of a bacterial cell that appear bright orange against a dark or green-fluorescing background when bound to fluorescent acridine orange stain.

    a. Cellulose and chitin
    b. Peptidoglycan layers
    c. Nucleic acids
    d. Mycolic acids

69. What is the most common causative agent of osteomyelitis when it is traumatically introduced to tissues and the bloodstream in a healthy individual?

    a. *Salmonella* spp.
    b. *Streptococcus aureus*
    c. *Brucella* spp.
    d. *Streptococcus agalactiae*

70. Which blood and bone marrow pathogen has the following virulence mechanisms that aid in the establishment and spread of infection?

    Antigenic lipopolysaccharide outer surface
    O-surface antigens
    Ability to survive extreme temperatures and pH levels

    a. *Salmonella* spp.
    b. *Streptococcus aureus*
    c. *Brucella* spp.
    d. *Streptococcus agalactiae*

71. What meningitis-causing agent is transmitted to humans via contaminated food and possesses internalin for access into host cells for intracellular growth and bacterial spread?

    a. *Listeria monocytogenes*
    b. *Escherichia coli*
    c. *Neisseria meningitidis*
    d. *Streptococcus pneumoniae*

72. What Gram-positive organism uses the following virulence mechanisms to establish and spread infections in body fluids and other normally sterile body sites?

    Alpha, beta, epsilon, iota, toxins
    A species-specific endotoxin
    Hemolysins, proteases, lipases, collagenase, hyaluronidase

    a. *Neisseria* spp.
    b. *Enterococcus*
    c. Beta-hemolytic *Streptococcus* spp.
    d. *Clostridium perfringens*

73. Three days after being admitted to the hospital, a patient presents with a fever and cough producing bloody sputum. The organism responsible establishes an infection and spreads via the following virulence mechanisms:

    Encapsulated with fimbriae
    Releases an inflammation inducing lipopolysaccharide endotoxin
    Iron-sequestering siderophores
    What organism is the cause of this hospital-acquired infection?

    a. *Legionella*
    b. *Klebsiella pneumoniae*
    c. *Mycobacterium tuberculosis*
    d. *Mycoplasma pneumoniae*

74. An infant presents with a fever, nasal congestion, and a severe cough that produces a high-pitched sound upon the intake of each breath. The following bacterial toxins aid in the establishment and spread of disease: PTx S2 and S3 adhere to epithelial cells and phagocytes, tracheal cytotoxin destroys ciliated respiratory epithelial cells, and the lethal toxin causes localized inflammation and tissue necrosis. What organism is the likely cause of the infection?

    a. *Corynebacterium diphtheriae*
    b. *Streptococcus pyogenes*
    c. *Bordetella pertussis*
    d. *Streptococcus pneumoniae*

75. *Helicobacter pylori* rapidly metabolizes urea to carbon dioxide and ammonia molecules. Which of the following detection methods applies this principle to indirectly confirm an active *H. pylori* infection?

    a. Urea breath test
    b. Polymerase chain reaction (PCR)
    c. IgG antibody serology
    d. Rapid urease test

76. _____ is an encapsulated, opportunistic anaerobe that produces beta-lactamase and causes infections in the skin, soft tissue, and bone if it is displaced from the gastrointestinal tract or introduced via soft-tissue trauma.

    a. *Pseudomonas aeruginosa*
    b. *Bacteroides fragilis*
    c. *Proteus mirabilis*
    d. *Prevotella* spp.

77. A male patient is seen by his healthcare provider for frequent and painful urination with a burning sensation and watery penile discharge. Suspecting acute urethritis caused by a sexually transmitted infection (STI), the provider submits a urine sample to the laboratory for testing. *Mycoplasma genitalium* is determined to be the causative pathogen. Which of the following methods of detection did the laboratory use to make this determination?

    a. Bright-orange appearance with fluorochrome acridine orange stain
    b. "Fried egg"-appearing colonies following four weeks of incubation
    c. Detection of the *tuf* gene via nucleic acid amplification testing (NAAT)
    d. Growth on sterol-enriched media at 35–37 °C in 95% nitrogen, 5% carbon

78. A patient exhibits the following symptoms: painful urination, pelvic pain, and increased vaginal discharge. Pili and IgA protease contain antiphagocytic properties and adhere to host mucosal cells for the establishment of the infection caused by which of the following organisms?

    a. *Neisseria gonorrhoeae*
    b. *Gardnerella vaginalis*
    c. *Treponema pallidum*
    d. *Chlamydia trachomatis*

79. A stool sample is submitted to the laboratory for a patient with unexplained diarrhea. A diagnosis of toxigenic *C. difficile* is confirmed by _____, which detects variable regions of the bacterial genome that express toxins A and B.

    a. 16s rRNA sequencing
    b. Toxin A/B enzyme immunoassays
    c. Glutamate dehydrogenase antigen tests
    d. PCR

80. What class of antibiotics binds to the peptidoglycan precursor of Gram-positive organisms, effectively inhibiting cell wall synthesis and causing cell death?

    a. Aminoglycoside
    b. Beta-lactam
    c. Macrolide
    d. Glycopeptide

81. A rectal swab is submitted to the laboratory for a patient admitted to the hospital. PCR testing is performed to screen for the _____ gene, which expresses antibiotic resistance in *Enterococci* colonizing the gastrointestinal tract.

    a. Beta-lactamase
    b. vanA
    c. Carbapenemase
    d. mecA

82. Select agents require the use of a biologic safety hood in the laboratory due to the highly infectious nature of aerosols produced during analysis. A technologist examines a sputum sample on the benchtop and later develops a fever, cough, chest pain, and difficulty breathing. The organism cultivated is identified as _____, due to its encapsulation, pili, acid phosphatase, and siderosomes.

    a. *Yersinia pestis*
    b. *Mycobacterium tuberculosis*
    c. *Bacillus anthracis*
    d. *Francisella tularensis*

83. An immunocompromised patient with symptoms of pneumonia submits a sputum sample to the laboratory. Following cultivation, an isolated culture colony is suspended in saline and the following procedure is performed:

    1. The suspension is fixed to a crystalline matrix and blasted with a laser.
    2. Molecules are vaporized without becoming fragmented or destroyed.
    3. Ionized molecules are separated based on their mass-to-charge ratio.
    4. Separated molecules are measured by the time elapsed between eluting and reaching the detector.

What is the next step in the process that allows for the determination of *Nocardia asteroides* as the organism responsible for the infection?

    a. An amplified target sequence is detected by attachment to chemiluminescent probes.
    b. Primers attach and amplify a new target strand created by restriction endonuclease.
    c. The molecular data produced are plotted onto a line graph and compared to a catalog of graphs of known organisms.
    d. Genetic sequences produced by variable regions are compared to sequences of known organisms.

84. Rifampin resistance is mediated by the _____ gene. Molecular detection of this gene provides pertinent information regarding antimicrobial treatment of active *M. tuberculosis* infections.

    a. RNA polymerase
    b. Gyrase B
    c. 65-kDa heat shock protein
    d. Catalase

85. Which of the following drug regimens is prescribed to treat infections caused by nontuberculous *Mycobacteria* organisms?

    a. Sulfonamide agent for 6–12 months
    b. Rifampin and ethambutol for 6–12 months
    c. Macrolide followed by rifampin and ethambutol for 6–18 months
    d. Sulfonamide agent and amikacin for 6–12 months

86. An abscess forms on a patient's arm at the site where they received a cut while gardening. The pathogen evaded phagocytosis and produced large amounts of catalase and hemolysins to establish the infection. What organism is most likely responsible?

    a. Nontuberculous *Mycobacteria*
    b. *Streptococcus aureus*
    c. *Nocardia* spp.
    d. *Streptococcus pyogenes*

87. An infection caused by _____ is usually diagnosed by macroscopically finding adult roundworms with curved or straight tails in a stool sample.

    a. *Taenia solium*
    b. *Diphyllobothrium latum*
    c. *Ascaris lumbricoides*
    d. *Enterobius vermicularis*

88. A sample cultured on Sabouraud dextrose agar produced white, smooth, mucoid colonies after 48 hours of incubation at 37 °C in 5% CO_2. Which fungal pathogen was cultivated?

    a. *Cryptococcus neoformans*
    b. *Histoplasma capsulatum*
    c. *Candida albicans*
    d. *Aspergillus fumigatus*

89. A bone marrow aspirate is submitted to the laboratory. Small, round to oval-shaped cells measuring 2–5 μm in diameter are observed intracellularly in the cytoplasm of mononuclear cells, indicating a possible *H. capsulatum* infection. Which of the following stains allows for this distinction?

    a. Acid fast
    b. Calcofluor white with potassium hydroxide (KOH)
    c. India ink
    d. Wright's

90. Culture of a sputum specimen produces the growth of a yeast-like organism. What biochemical test can be performed on the isolate for rapid differentiation between *C. albicans* and *C. neoformans*?

a. Germ tube test
b. Urease test
c. Capsular antigen latex agglutination
d. India ink stain

91. A urine sample is sent to your laboratory for confirmation testing following a positive screen for barbiturates. The "gold standard" methodology for drug confirmation is performed as follows:

Step 1:
A sample is introduced to a capillary column in the stationary phase.
Molecules are separated based on their individual chemical properties and affinity for the column.
Molecules of each substance elute off the column at different speeds and migrate to step 2.
Step 2:
Molecules are ionized via fragmentation or electron loss.
Ionized molecules are focused into a beam, increasing their kinetic energy, and then they pass through a magnetic field.

What action takes place next for the detection and quantification of drug and drug metabolite molecules?

a. A color produced is compared to known concentrations.
b. Molecules migrate in varying distances and patterns.
c. A visible immunogenic compound forms.
d. Ions deflect at varying speeds and angles.

92. Principles determined for the appropriate conduct of an individual or group in the workplace are known as what type of ethics in healthcare?

a. Beneficence
b. Personal
c. Professional
d. Medical

93. In accordance with HIPAA, which of the following is NOT an appropriate instance for laboratory staff to access protected health information?

a. Sharing patient health records with a family member without prior consent from the patient
b. Providing patient demographics to public health departments in regard to reportable diseases
c. Accessing a family member's laboratory results when necessary for a job-related task
d. Accessing previous diagnosis and laboratory reports for correlation with current laboratory results

94. Which of the following is an example of the advantages of integrating automation into the postanalytical phase of laboratory processes?

a. The laboratory information system (LIS) generates a unique account number for each admission that is linked to the patient's medical record number.
b. Bar coded samples on the analyzer are linked to test requisitions in the LIS, and the appropriate test is performed on each sample.
c. Normal test results are automatically verified by the LIS through mathematical algorithms based on laboratory policies.
d. Laboratory test orders entered into the LIS automatically generate requisitions and specimen bar codes.

95. Which if the following is an example of an error that occurs during the analytical phase of a laboratory process?

a. A sample tube collected for coagulation testing was not filled with the appropriate volume of blood.
b. Hemoglobin A1C calibrations must be done every 30 days. The technologist runs a patient sample for an A1C with a calibration that is 32 days old.
c. The technologist manually enters laboratory results for patient A into the LIS under the test requisition for patient B.
d. Chemistry reagents that must be stored at 2–8 °C are left in their shipping container overnight and reach a temperature of 20 °C.

Answer Key and Explanations

1. D: All of the above. Receiving cannot accession a specimen without:

- A label that clearly states the patient's name, collection date, doctor's name and contact information, specimen type, and test required.
- An uncontaminated, valid requisition bearing the doctor's signature, patient's billing information, and pertinent information (acute or convalescent phase, antibiotic use, fever, or traveler).
- Intact specimen container.
- Correct media type or preservative used for the specimen type.
- Same-day collection date, or preincubated at room temperature or subcultivated, and then vented, to prevent false-negatives of nonfermentative species.
- If the specimen does not meet these conditions, call the doctor's office and get the missing information. Discard the specimen if you cannot obtain full information, and inform the doctor's office that recollection is required.

2. A: 120 gallons of class I, II, and IIIA liquids. Choice A complies with fire safety standards. Class IA, IB, and IC are flammables. Class II, IIIA, and IIIB are combustibles. No more than 120 gallons of class I, II, and IIIA liquids can be stored in a lab fridge, and of those, no more than 60 gallons may be class I and II. Do not locate more than three storage cabinets in one fire area. No more than 50% of the flammables can be stored for teaching. Use DOT-approved glass, metal, or polyethylene containers no larger than 1.1 gallons (4 L).

3. A: How probable it is a patient will develop a disease, and its etiology. A is correct because disease incidence measures how prevalent a disease is among a given population in a specific place, over a specific time. Incidence predicts how probable it is a patient will develop a disease, and its etiology (likely cause). B,C, and D are incorrect because they refer to a related concept called predicted values, which estimate how likely a test result is to be right or wrong, given certain variables, such as the patient's age, occupation, race, income, how long the symptoms have lasted, and if there is fever.

4. B: Only applies if absorbance is between 0.1 and 1.0. B is correct because Beer's law states absorbance is proportional to the concentration of a solution, but Beer's law only applies if absorbance is between 0.1 and 1.0. Different substances absorb different light wavelengths, so a spectrophotometer (Spec-20) compares the intensity of light entering a sample and exiting from it (percent transmittance) to find the concentration of the sample. A completely transparent sample has 100% transmittance. A completely opaque sample has 0% transmittance. Visible spectrum light ranges from 440 nm to 700 nm.

5. C: Presumptive identification. C is correct. Note the color, outline (circular, rhizoid, or wavy), elevation (convex, flat, or raised), and translucency (opaque, translucent, or transparent) for presumptive identification. Differential identification means naming bacteria according to their headspace gases and volatile compounds they release as they grow on media, with a spectrometer (microDMx). Adanson's numerical taxonomy (phonetics) ranks microorganisms according to how similar they are genetically and morphologically. Closely related bacteria form a cluster, which is classified into objective, repeatable taxa. *TaqMan*, SWOrRD, and *MicroSeq* are quick screening kits. They are not as accurate as cultures but are quicker when time is critical. Polymerase chain

113

reaction (PCR) in quick kits amplifies the genetic material, and then the 1450 base pair region of the 16S rDNA gene is sequenced by electrophoresis.

6. C: Both a and b. The US Occupational Safety and Health Administration (OSHA) sets the standards for proper hand washing, wearing gloves, bagging specimens in biohazard bags, and disposing of needles and lancets in a sharps safe container. Visit http://www.osha.gov regularly to find updates. OSHA requires phlebotomists to glove before every venipuncture as part of standard (universal) precautions for bloodborne pathogens. Only in a volunteer blood donation center does OSHA allow for ungloved venipunctures, providing the phlebotomist is experienced and not a trainee. The phlebotomist must agree not to glove. The employer must provide gloves if the phlebotomist wants them. If the phlebotomist is allergic to latex or powdered gloves, the employer must provide hypoallergenic or unpowdered gloves, liners, or barrier cream. The phlebotomist must glove if her skin is broken or burnt, or has a rash. If the patient is combative or likely to have a reaction, then the phlebotomist must glove. Employers must reevaluate the no-glove policy periodically to see if it continues to be a low-risk option. Whenever contact with blood is likely, such as during infant heel pricks, gloves are required.

7. B: Toxicology. Serology/Immunology studies antibodies in the liquid part of blood. Cytology studies cells for cancer, such as Pap smears. Endocrinology studies hormones, such as diabetes and acromegaly.

8. C: Normal hemoglobin. Hemoglobin electrophoresis differentiates hemoglobin into normal HbA and normal HbA_2, or abnormal HbS in sickle cell patients, or HbC in hemolytic anemia patients, or HbF in a fetus or newborn.

9. D: All of the above. Doctors, nurses, social workers, chiropractors, law officers, daycare staff, clergy, teachers, and psychologists were declared mandatory reporters in 1996. This means they must report certain occurrences or suspicions orally to the proper authorities within 24 hours and follow up with a written report within 48 hours. For example, a doctor must report STD or TB to Public Health to prevent an epidemic. Caregivers have the right to know the patient's diagnosis if it puts them at risk for infection or assault. Suspicion of child abuse, exploitation, or neglect is reported to Child Protective Services under the Child Abuse Prevention and Treatment Act (CAPTA). Each state has an abuse hotline. Many states require *anyone* who has reasonable cause to report child or elder abuse or face civil liability. You must know the law of the state in which you practice.

10. A: Sensitivity. Sensitivity (recall rate) measures how many times a test produces true-positive results, which indicates patients probably have a disease, compared with the gold standard test for that particular illness. Sensitivity allows early detection of disease and prevents epidemics. Divide the number of patients who definitely have the disease and test positive by the total patients tested who have the disease (including those who tested false-negative), and multiply by 100 to obtain the percentage sensitivity. Specificity measures how many times a test produces true-negative results, meaning patients probably do not have a disease, compared with the gold standard test for that particular illness. Specificity is important for cancer chemotherapy and other toxic treatments. Aliquot is dividing a solution into equal parts. Aliquot allows very expensive reagents or drugs, and blood samples that are below scale, to be used efficiently. Circadian rhythm is a normal daily flow that affects hormones, which are normally higher in the morning than in the afternoon.

11. C: Green, gray, and marbled SST blood collection tubes. Hematology requires mostly lavender, light blue, and black tubes. Blood Bank and Public Health require red, pink, and yellow tubes. Toxicology requires navy, purple, and brown tubes. If you draw the wrong color tube, it contains an inappropriate anticoagulant, and the test will be invalidated.

12. A: BUN to Creatinine ratio between 15:1 and 20:1. Blood urea nitrogen (BUN) and creatinine are waste products of protein metabolism, measured in kidney function tests performed with a 24-hour urine. If the kidneys do not filter properly, creatinine output in the urine decreases, and creatine blood levels increase. High creatinine (more than 1.5 mg/dL) and BUN (more than 20 mg/dL) means the patient has a kidney disease (e.g., glomerulonephritis, pyelonephritis, stones, tubular necrosis, tumors). BUN and creatinine must be in correct proportion for optimal health. ALP and AST are liver function tests. Amylase is a pancreas test.

13. D: All of the above. Newborn jaundice is different from adult jaundice. Babies have more red blood cells and reticulocytes than adults do. Babies have immature livers that are not yet efficient at breaking down bilirubin. Adult jaundice is usually from hepatitis or cirrhosis of the liver. Erythroblastosis fetalis means the baby's Rh factor is incompatible with his mother's Rh, leading to hemolytic disease of the newborn. Kernicterus means the bilirubin is greater than 5 mg/dL, resulting in hemolytic anemia if not treated with phototherapy (blue lights). Physiologic jaundice occurs in breastfed babies released from the hospital too early and without a vitamin K injection, but resolves in a week with adequate fluids.

14. B: Triglycerides. Anions are negatively charged ions of chloride and bicarbonate. Cholesterol is lipids from animal sources that climb after a fatty meal. An eluent is a solvent used for chromatography.

15. C: Protein electrophoresis. The serum proteins test includes total protein, albumin, and globulin. Ascites is swelling of the abdomen from extra fluid in the peritoneum, resulting from end-stage diseases of the heart, kidney, liver, ovary, and pancreas. When serum proteins make the doctor suspect one of these diseases, the doctor follows up with protein electrophoresis. Four globulin fractionations are added to the total protein and albumin: alpha-1 globulin, alpha-2 globulin, beta globulin, and gamma globulin. Electrophoresis patterns and the patient's history of drug use help pinpoint the diagnosis, which may extend to rheumatoid arthritis, muscle tumors, and immune deficiencies. Bilirubin is the brownish-red bile pigment from broken down blood cells in the liver.

16. A: Alcoholism, hypothyroidism, cardioversion, or clofibrate use. Cardiac enzymes elevate soon after a heart attack, but that is not the only possible root cause. CPK elevates in alcoholism; cardiac catheterization; stroke; clofibrate use; electric shock applied during resuscitation; low thyroid hormone and high thyroid-stimulating hormone; and after surgery. B and D refer to situations that cause AST enzyme to rise. C refers to situations that cause LDH enzyme to rise.

17. D: Cushing syndrome. Cortisol is an adrenal stress hormone that is normally higher around 8:00 in the morning (6–28 mcg/dL) and lower at 4:00 in the afternoon (2–12 mcg/dL). The fluctuation is a normal diurnal variation. Cushing syndrome patients have sustained high cortisol. Addison's disease patients have chronically low cortisol levels, diagnosed by a 24-hour urine test for 17-hydroxycorticosteroids. Abnormal cortisol levels also appear in thyroid and pituitary gland disease, obesity, and cancer, and when steroids, diuretics, or birth control pills are used, but it is not the same pattern as Cushing syndrome. B refers to atrial natriuretic factor (ANF), produced by the heart's atria during volume overload and high blood pressure.

18. B: Hyponatremia, often from vomiting and diarrhea, furosemide, or Addison's disease. Hyponatremia results from too much water and not enough salt in the bloodstream. Hyponatremia often presents as a urine sample with a specific gravity (SG) lower than the normal 1.015–1.025 and closer to the SG of water (1.000). Hypernatremia refers to too much salt in the bloodstream, which increases SG above 1.025. Hyperkalemia and hypokalemia refer to the level of potassium, not sodium.

19. A: Rise 6 hours after heart attack, peak in 18 hours, and return to baseline in 3 days. CPK is the first enzyme to rise following a heart attack, so doctors measure it before the other cardiac enzymes. If creatine kinase-MB (CK-MB) rises, it means the heart sustained severe damage. B. refers to the response of AST to a heart attack. C refers to the response of LDH to a heart attack. D does not apply because alpha-fetoprotein (AFP) is used to find liver disease, testicular cancer, and birth defects.

20. B: Less than 7.20. pH stands for percentage of hydrogen. A blood pH test is performed with arterial blood gasses to determine if the patient has acidosis or alkalosis. The blood must be kept in a narrow range of pH from 7.35–7.45, so answer A would be low normal. Answer C, 80–100 torr, refers to normal percentage of oxygen. D is incorrect because an abnormal PSA result for prostate cancer is unrelated to blood pH.

21. A: 120 days. A normal erythrocyte (red blood cell [RBC]) lives for four months. When it wears out, the spleen destroys it and the liver converts it to bilirubin, which the gallbladder stores as bile and the digestive system uses to break down dietary fats. Old red blood cells puff into a sphere, rather than retaining their original barbell-shape. Changing shape makes them fragile and inflexible. Babies have 4.8–7.2 million RBCs per cubic millimeter of blood. Adult males have 4–6 million, and adult females 4–5 million RBCs. Pregnant women have lower RBC counts.

22. D: Rouleaux formation. Normal red blood cells settle slowly when standing in a test tube: males 0–15 millimeters per hour; females 0–20 mm/h; children 0–10 mm/h; elderly patients 5–10 mm/h more. A low sedimentation rate indicates hemorrhage. A high sedimentation rate indicates cells are heavier and falling quicker than normal, usually from inflammatory diseases, parasite infection, cell death, heavy metal poisoning, or toxemia of pregnancy. However, cold agglutinins also make red blood cells adhere to each other in a Rouleaux formation when they are chilled.

23. C: Leukocyte alkaline phosphatase (LAP). Hematologists use LAP stain to highlight neutrophils when the patient has many white blood cells but not leukemia (leukemic reaction). Microbiologists use periodic acid-Schiff (PAS) to stain carbohydrates, collagen, fibrin, and mucin purple. Sudan black B (SBB) is specifically for acute leukemia patients; it helps to differentiate between immature cells by staining lipids in myeloid leukemia that are absent in lymphoid leukemia. LPCB is mixed with 10% potassium hydroxide (KOH) to identify fungus.

24. D: Both a and c. Make a bone marrow slide with a battlement technique so the review is more standardized, with even cell distribution. Wedge push technique (feathered end) causes the white cells to pool unevenly on the slide. On the side edges and in the feather of a wedge push slide, you will find concentrated pockets of eosinophils, monocytes, and segmented neutrophils. Small lymphocytes concentrate in the center of the slide.

25. A: Phase I problems. Phase I of coagulation happens in the first 3–5 minutes after an injury, when the platelets mobilize. Factor III distress call is sent in phase II, not phase I. Factor VIII deficiency is the problem that causes hemophilia. Fibrinolysis occurs when the injured site is plugged with a blood clot and plasminogen changes to plasmin.

26. B: Lupus inhibitor antibody (LA). Hematologists use phospholipid in PT and PTT tests to check how fast a patient clots. The normal range for PTT is 60–70 seconds. Lupus inhibitor antibody (LA) acts against the phospholipid and falsely extends clotting time. LA is implicated in miscarriages, rheumatoid arthritis, lupus, Reynaud syndrome, and thromboembolism. Platelet antibody testing is only appropriate if the patient has purpura and hemoglobinuria. Intrinsic factor is incorrect; it is the stomach's ability to produce B_{12} to prevent pernicious anemia.

27. B: Fungal serology titer of more than 1:32 that increases x4 or more 3 weeks later. First, gently scrape suspected fungus off the patient's skin. Mix two drops of 10% potassium hydroxide (KOH) and one drop of LPCB on a glass slide, cover it, and warm it to observe budding yeasts. Add a drop of calcofluor white before warming to see fluorescent infected tissue. Put a drop of India ink on a wet mount to see clear cryptococcal capsules. Confirm the microscopic exam with fungal serology when you test the skin scraping and again in three weeks. The doctor may follow up by ordering latex serology for cryptococcal antigen to find meningitis, complement fixation for coccidiomycosis and histoplasmosis, and immunodiffusion for blastomycosis.

28. A: Plasmacrit test (PCT) and rapid plasma reagin (RPR) test. The old screening test for syphilis is VDRL, which measures *Treponema pallidum* antibodies by flocculation reaction to the diphosphatidyl glycerol in ox heart extract. However, VDRL misses cases of syphilis that are less than four weeks old, and half of cases that are in the late stages. VDRL is not very sensitive, and often gives a false-positive result for patients with the following conditions: pregnancy, hepatitis, HIV, leprosy, lupus (SLE), Lyme disease, malaria, mononucleosis, pneumonia, rheumatic fever, or rheumatoid arthritis. PCT and RCR are less likely to be confounded, and since they require less blood, are replacing VDRL. ELISA confirms syphilis infection by identifying the specific antibodies. FTA-ABS is 100% accurate for secondary syphilis, but it is expensive, and the patient will always test positive once infected. Captia is required to confirm RPR. Cold agglutinins increase in children with congenital syphilis.

29. D: Dilute 1 mL of serum with 1 mL of saline. You must know how to dilute to perform a titer, which measures how many times a blood sample must be diluted with saline before an antibody can no longer be found in it. First, check the antibody/antigen reaction against the controls with undiluted serum. To prevent blood clotting (Rouleaux formation) during dilution, warm the blood and saline to body temperature (37 °C) for 10 minutes before diluting. Dilute 1 mL of serum with 1 mL of saline for a dilution of ½, or 1:2. Pipette off 1 mL of this dilution into an aliquot tube. Add 1 mL of saline, and it becomes a 1:4 dilution. If you dilute up to 1:32 and get no reaction, the end-point titer is 16.

30. A: Guinea pig, cow, and horse. Monospot heterophile antibodies test confirms an early infection of mononucleosis, caused by Epstein-Barr virus. If the infection is older than 9 weeks, then the doctor orders EBV antibody test. On a glass slide, mix a drop of the patient's blood with guinea pig kidney antigen to absorb Forssman antibodies. Add beef red blood stroma to absorb non-Forssman antibodies. Mix with horse blood. Guinea pig agglutination means the patient has early mononucleosis. Beef should not agglutinate. Monospot can be false-negative on children younger than 10, or before two weeks of infection. B, C, and D are not applicable to Monospot.

31. C: Both syphilis and HIV. Patients coinfected with HIV and syphilis are immunosuppressed. When performing a titer to find antibodies in an HIV/syphilitic, beware prozone phenomenon. The coinfected patient's undiluted serum may produce a false-negative result because it does not agglutinate. Alternatively, it may show very little agglutination at low dilutions, but agglutinates more at higher dilutions because of excess antibodies. Monospot is used to find EBV mononucleosis. Reynaud disease is characterized by rouleaux formation and high cold agglutinin titers. IgG occurs in patients who are convalescing from mononucleosis.

117

32. D: Both a and b. *RhoGAM* is the brand name for Rh immunoglobulin. It is administered to Rh-women who acquired anti-D antibodies from a previous blood transfusion or pregnancy. The infant and father do not receive *RhoGAM* at all. If there is a live birth, the mother gets 300 mcg of *RhoGAM* during week 26–28 of her pregnancy, and again before her infant is 3 days old. If the pregnancy miscarries before week 13 or is aborted, then the mother gets a lower dose of 50 mcg of *MICRhoGAM*. If the miscarriage or abortion happens after week 13, use *RhoGAM*.

33. A: Eosinophilia, hypocalcemia, leukopenia, and pancytopenia may occur. The first lab sign of a mild transfusion reaction is the oxyhemoglobin dissociation curve shifts left. Later, the number of eosinophils will increase and the calcium level will drop. Finally, white blood cells will decrease, and then all blood cells will decrease. Minimize the chance of transfusion reaction by washing the donor's red blood cells in sterile normal saline before transfusion. If the doctor anticipates a mild transfusion reaction, he/she may give antihistamines to the patient before transfusion, and may order the removal of white cells from the bag of blood by a Sepacell R-500 leukocyte reduction filter. Irradiated blood products prevent fatal transfusion-associated graft-versus-host disease (TA-GVHD). The safest way for a patient to prepare for elective surgery is to bank his own blood for transfusion (autologous donation).

34. C: No A or B antigens and both anti-A and anti-B antibodies. Type O- blood is the universal donor because it has no A or B antigens, or Rh+ antibodies. If there is no time to crossmatch a trauma patient, then O– blood is given without compatibility testing to prevent death. A routine type and cross takes 45 minutes and the delay could be fatal.

35. B: Trauma patient with hemoglobin of 5 g/dL. Blood Bank triages patients in the following priority sequence: (1) emergency trauma victims with isovolemic anemia from hemorrhage; (2) surgical patients who lose more than 3 cups of blood; (3) regular users of coagulation factors. If you anticipate a blood shortage because of a massive trauma, then contact the nurse manager as soon as possible. The surgical team may decide to cancel elective surgery, or delay it until the patient is medically treated to reduce anemia. If surgery must proceed, the surgical team may consider the following blood conservation methods if you warn them ahead of time: erythropoietin, autologous donations, or hemodilution before surgery; cell savers, hypotension, electrocautery, and lasers during surgery; and administering antifibrinolytics after surgery.

36. D: All of the above. A type and cross is very time-consuming (45 minutes) and must meet very specific safety standards to avoid a transfusion reaction. All of the following conditions must be met:

- Specimens labeled at the patient's bedside with full name or the emergency department identification number; initials are unacceptable. Specimens must not have pink serum. Donor blood must not be clotted, fatty, or contaminated.
- Patient wears an identification band, which is checked at collection *and* transfusion times. The band must not be taped to the bed. The patient's name and a unique identification number (Blood Bank identification number, hospital number, health insurance number, or unique lifetime identifier) must appear on the band, in case there is a patient with a similar name.
- Requisitions must bear the collector's and identifier's names, collection date and time (in case antibodies develop), the ordering doctor's name, the amount and type of blood requested, the patient's date of birth (if known), relevant patient history (e.g., pregnant and bleeding; signs of transfusion reaction).

37. A: Midstream urine collection (MSU). MSU is required to diagnose cystitis and pyelitis accurately. Witnessed collection is only required for drug testing. 24-hour urines are for hormone tests. Random urine may have contamination, so while it is suitable for chemistry, random urine is inaccurate for microbiology. Collect midstream urine any time of day, in a sterile, lidded container. Your microbiologist may want the patient to use a benzalkonium chloride wipe before collection. Without a wipe, the sample is not a clean catch. Do not touch the inside of the container, as it contaminates the specimen and produces a false-positive.

38. A: Cell count, glucose and protein, gram stain and culture, virology/mycology/cytology. Only a physician can collect cerebrospinal fluid (CSF) from a lumbar puncture. The MLT just prepares a collection tray and assists as ordered. The tray must contain the following: iodine prep; alcohol prep; 3 cc of 1% lidocaine; 25g, 5/8" needle; 22g, 1.5" needle; atraumatic spinal needle (to prevent postcollection headache); syringe; four sterile red stoppered tubes; 4x4 gauze; sponge forceps; sterile towels; small basin; and a Band-Aid. The physician collects the fluid between L3 and L4 in the patient's spine and hands you the tubes. Label one tube each for cell count, glucose and protein, gram stain and culture, and virology/mycology/cytology. You only need a fifth tube if the physician wants globulin immunoelectrophoresis, which is rare. C and D tests are included in A, and it is unnecessary to requisition them separately.

39. C: Pyorrhea and Lemierre syndrome. The pathogenic phyla are xenobacteria, cyanobacteria, firmicutes, flavobacteria, fusobacteria, planctomycetes, proteobacteria, spirochaetes, and verrucomicrobia. Planctomycetes causes chlamydia and pneumonia. Spirochaetes cause Lyme disease. Proteobacteria causes stomach ulcers. Firmicutes cause food poisoning. Fusobacteria cause pockets of pus in the gums that can break off into septic blood clots in the jugular vein of the neck. The septic clots can travel to cause abscesses in distant parts of the body, such as the brain, joints, kidney, and liver. Lemierre syndrome from gum disease was common until the discovery of antibiotics.

40. D: Löwenstein-Jensen (LJ) egg. TB is a fussy bacterium to grow in the lab and requires egg media. Tinsdale is used to find *C. diphtheria*. Sheep blood is used to find slow-growing anaerobic bacteria. MYW is used to find *Legionella* pneumonia. It is important for the MLT to know what type of infection the doctor suspects, so the correct media can be used for culture. Failure to pick the correct media may result in a false-negative and the disease will go undiagnosed.

41. B: 10x. To find parasites such as worms, set the microscope's magnification to 10x. Parasites often cause bleeding, so set the microscope to 40x to find the blood cells. Higher powers are unnecessary to view animal parasites and count cells, and would just slow down the MLT's reading of the slide. Calibrate the ocular micrometer every time a new technician is hired, each time you change optics, and annually thereafter.

42. A: Crypto (*Cryptosporidium parvum*). In the United States, the lab technician is required by law to report the following nine parasites to Public Health authorities if they are found in patient samples: *Cryptosporidium parvum, Cyclospora cayetanensis, Entamoeba histolytica,* hematoxylin, *Giardia duodenalis, Plasmodium falciparum, Taenia, Trichinella spiralis,* and *Enterobius vermicularis.* Hookworm, tapeworm, and pinworm are very common infestations and do not need to be reported. Your lab must provide reference slides or a parasite atlas for you to compare against the patients' specimens. Keep positive specimens in your lab for at least one year, either as a permanently stained slide, or as a preserved stool sample that is safely stored. Public Health may order them for examination.

43. D: Wet mount fresh, liquid stool with LPCB stain. *Giardia lamblia* is a parasite that lives in the small intestine of humans who consume contaminated food or water. *Giardia* causes traveler's diarrhea. *Giardia* cysts are activated by stomach acid and become trophozoites. The MLT can get the patient to swallow a string for several hours and then examine it for trophozoites, but many patients are uncooperative and prefer to leave a stool sample instead. To prepare the wet mount, strain well-formed stool. Concentrate it in the centrifuge at 2000 rpm for 4 minutes in a conical tube. Ream the tube with a wooden stick. Add 10% formalin. Make a tan suspension. You should be able to read a newspaper through the slide. Examine microscopically at 10x for parasites and 40x for blood. Use an ocular micrometer to measure parasites. Mix stool with PVA plastic powder to glue it onto the slide before permanent staining with iodine or *Snap n' Stain*.

44. B: One year. Parasites are a serious Public Health issue. It is important to prevent parasites acquired in foreign countries from spreading through the American populace. Even though you check your patient's specimen against reference slides or a parasite atlas, you could miss rare species or misidentify the parasite in its different stages of development. A Public Health official has the right to check your slide for one year after initial testing. To ensure your test is accurate, use positive and negative controls to check your antigens every time you receive a new shipment and every month thereafter. Use the right stain for the right specimen. Refrigerate stool within three hours of receiving it, if you do not have time to fix it with preservative.

45. D: Mycology specimens. The MLT uses a Wood's lamp to help identify fungus on the patient's skin before collecting it. Fungus will fluoresce bright lime green under the Wood's light, so the MLT will find it easily and can scrape it off with a tongue depressor into a sterile container for testing. Malaria parasites are found in blood smears. Public Health specimens are usually blood serology or stool for parasites. Toxicology specimens are usually red, navy, or purple stoppered blood tubes for drugs or heavy metals.

46. D: Nitrites. There is a nitrite pad on an *N-Multistix* for routine urinalysis. Some bacteria eat nitrates in urine, and shed nitrites as a waste product. *E. coli* is one of the bacteria detectable by nitrites in urine. However, not finding nitrites does not mean there is no infection. For example, strep is a very serious and common kidney infection, but does not produce nitrites. Leukocytes indicate an infection in a person with a healthy immune system, but an immunosuppressed patient may not produce leukocytes in urine. Protein indicates kidney damage, but it is not necessarily from an infection. Ketones are a byproduct of fat metabolism that appear in diabetic patients and crash dieters.

47. A: Testicular cancer. Do not assume that the doctor filled out the wrong name and sex on the requisition if you receive a request for a pregnancy test on a man. A pregnancy test looks for the hormone beta-human chorionic gonadotropin (hCG). A pregnant woman excretes beta-hCG 10 days after conceiving a child. However, a male with carcinoma of the testicles also excretes this same pregnancy hormone. Normal males never excrete beta-hCG. If your patient had an orchiectomy (removal of the testicles) but is still excreting beta-hCG in a follow-up test, then metastasized cancer is present. The doctor must remove it surgically, or with radiation or chemotherapy. Prostatitis would produce leukocytes but not hCG. Cryptorchidism is undescended testicles, which can lead to cancer in later life. Peyronie disease is a bent penis from scar tissue, and does not produce hCG.

48. D: 750–2,000 mL. A patient should produce at least 500 mL (2 cups) of urine each and every day. Ideally, a patient should produce 750 mL (3 cups) to 2,000 mL (5 cups) of urine to maintain good health. If the patient has vomiting and diarrhea, or an enlarged prostate gland or severe infection, or uses too much medication, then he will produce scanty urine (oliguria). Some of the drug overdoses that decrease urinary output are anticholinergics, methotrexate, and diuretics. Patients whose kidneys are failing have anuria, which strictly interpreted means absence of urine, but they actually produce 100 mL or less of urine per day. Patients who have diabetes insipidus or diabetes mellitus often produce far too much urine (3½ quarts or more). They are very thirsty and may drink more than a gallon of fluid per day (more than 12 glasses). The antidepressant lithium is one drug that can cause frequent urination as an adverse effect.

49. C: Gout. Patients with gout have extreme pain in their great toes due to needles of uric acid crystals that form around their joints. Patients with struvite crystals in their urine have bacterial infections. Patients with tyrosine or cystine crystals in their urine may be poisoned or have a serious metabolic disorder. Patients with phosphate or calcium oxalate crystals in their urine have too much parathyroid hormone or malabsorption. Crystals do not appear in healthy urine.

50. C: Hematuria and uroliths. Polycystic kidney disease is an inherited disorder that produces bloody urine and kidney stones. It is the most common inherited disease in the United States, and it is the fourth leading cause of kidney failure. Cysts may also appear in the patient's liver, but do not produce cirrhosis or hepatitis. Destruction of the kidney does eventually produce high blood pressure, but the PKD patient is a poor candidate for a bypass graft because of abnormal heart valves. The patient may develop abnormal pockets in the intestine that fill with hard stool (diverticulosis); however, they seldom produce severe bleeding. Melena is a tarry, black stool caused by internal bleeding, and hematochezia is red stools caused by heavy bleeding.

51. C: Platelet refractoriness is the inability to achieve a desired platelet count following the transfusion of platelets that can be caused by immune or nonimmune processes. Incompatibilities between patient and donor human leukocyte antigens (HLAs) can cause the immune system to create alloantibodies against the donor platelets. **Class I HLAs** are present on the surface of platelets and nucleated cells, and they are most often responsible for immune-mediated platelet refractoriness. **Class II HLAs** do not cause alloimmunization against platelet HLAs because they are found on the surface of lymphocytes, activated T lymphocytes, monocytes, macrophages, and dendritic cells. Platelets do not express **Rh antigens** on their surface, and the negligible amount of red blood cells present in apheresis platelets cannot cause anti-D alloimmunization in Rh-negative patients. Transfusion of mismatched **ABO** platelets is capable of causing a decreased response to platelet therapy; however, this outcome is not due to platelet alloantibodies and is considered a non-immune-mediated cause of platelet refractoriness.

52. B: Neutralization and inhibition techniques are performed to allow otherwise masked alloantibodies to bind to reagent red blood cells for detection. Reagent serum containing soluble antigens to Lewis, P1, Sd^a, and Chido and Rodgers antibodies is added to a sample and binds with the antibodies, inhibiting their ability to bind with reagent red blood cells and neutralizing their ability to react. **Elution** techniques determine antibody specificity by breaking the antigen–antibody bond on patient red blood cells and releasing the antibody into a solution. **Inactivation** methods use reagents and enzymes to destroy, weaken, and remove antigens, antibodies, or complement from patient red blood cells for allo- and autoantibody identification. **Adsorption** techniques use patient or reagent red blood cells to remove autoantibodies or separate multiple antibodies to determine the following: underlying alloantibodies previously masked by autoantibodies, the presence of red blood cell surface antigens, and confirmation of antibody specificity.

53. C: High-performance liquid chromatography methodologies dissolve substances in a liquid solution and apply high pressure to force the substances through a gradient for qualitative and quantitative detection of hemoglobin variants. Hemoglobinopathies and glycosylated hemoglobin molecules will separate based on their ionic reactions with exchange cations on the gradient's surface. **Flow cytometry** detects and categorizes substances based on the light scatter produced by particles as they are passed through a laser beam. **Gas chromatography-mass spectrometry** separates molecules based on their chemical properties and their affinity for the cylindrical column that they pass through and detects them based on their mass-to-charge ratio. **Liquid chromatography-tandem mass spectrometry** combines the separation of particles based on the interactions of their mobile and stationary phases with detection and quantification by dual mass spectrometry.

54. A: Acquired coagulation inhibitors are monoclonal antibodies that act against clotting factors and phospholipids that can form in response to the following situations: use of pooled or commercial clotting factors for the treatment of bleeding disorders, malignancy, pregnancy, and autoimmune diseases. **Natural coagulation inhibitors** circulate in the bloodstream to balance the hemostatic effect of clotting factors and reduce the risk of unnecessary clot formation. Circulating acquired inhibitors will decrease a patient's ability to clot properly, which causes elevated PT, aPTT, and fibrinogen degradation product results. Acquired inhibitors are also indicated by increased monoclonal antibodies that act against clotting factors, whereas naturally occurring inhibitors do not. Detection of **factors V and X deficiencies** begins with prolonged PT and PTT results but is followed by a TT and mixing studies.

55. D: A patient presenting with a prolonged PT and aPTT will require further coagulation testing to determine the cause of these results. First, a TT test is performed to determine if heparin therapy is the reason for the prolonged coagulation results. A positive TT result indicates that a patient is receiving heparin therapy, whereas a negative TT result rules this out as a cause. Following a negative or normal TT result, **mixing studies** are performed on patient plasma to distinguish whether factor deficiencies or coagulation inhibitors are causing decreased clotting activity. **Lupus anticoagulant** and **factor assays** are performed only after lupus anticoagulant or factor deficiencies have been identified by mixing studies as the cause of the initial prolonged PT and aPTT results. **von Willebrand factor assays are** not indicated in this instance because von Willebrand disease does not present with prolonged PT results.

56. C: Factor assays use functional clotting methodologies to determine the activity of and confirm suspected deficiencies of individual coagulation factors. Serial dilutions of patient plasma and factor-deficient reagent plasma are prepared, and the PT or PTT of each dilution is measured and plotted on a line graph. Factor activity is determined by the amount of correction measured with each serial dilution. **PT-based assays** determine the function of the following factors from the extrinsic and common pathways: V, **VII, X**, and **II. PTT assays** are performed to evaluate intrinsic and common pathway factors including **VIII**, IX, XI, and XII. **Russell's viper venom (RVV)** contains the enzymes required to specifically activate factors V and **X**. RVV assays record the time it takes for a clot to form in factor-deficient plasma following a 30 second incubation at 37 °C and the addition of RVV and calcium chloride. Results obtained for each dilution are plotted on a line graph and compared to a standard curve for factor X activity.

57. B: A defect or dysfunction of factor VIII: von Willebrand factor (vWF) is responsible for **von Willebrand disease**. In response to an injury, vWF protein binds to exposed collagen and platelet glycoproteins to aid in platelet aggregation and adhesion. PT and platelet counts are normal in patients with von Willebrand disease because the extrinsic pathway of the coagulation cascade and platelet production are not influenced by vWF. Normal or elevated PTT results and decreased factor VIII activity indicate the dysfunction of factor VIII in the intrinsic coagulation pathway. Ristocetin platelet aggregation studies evaluate the function of vWF because ristocetin acts on vWF to induce its binding to platelet glycoproteins. Decreased platelet aggregation in the presence of ristocetin indicates vWF disease.

Hemophilia A and **factor IX deficiency** are both disorders of the intrinsic pathway in the coagulation cascade; therefore, the PTT results will be elevated whereas the PT results will maintain normal values. Platelet aggregation is not affected by deficiencies of factors VII and IX.

Disseminated intravascular coagulation (DIC) is caused by a dysregulation of fibrinolysis that can occur in response to various underlying conditions. Abnormal clotting in DIC consumes large amounts of platelets and clotting factors in the blood vessels, causing a decrease of them in circulation and excessive bleeding elsewhere in the body. Due to the consumption of these components intravascularly, DIC is indicated by prolonged PT and PTT results and decreased platelet counts.

58. A: Agonists are used during platelet aggregation studies to replicate and evaluate the response that they elicit from platelets at various stages of the coagulation process. In vivo, **collagen** exposed during an injury will bind to glycoprotein Ib (GpIb), induce the release of granules, and begin platelet plug formation with platelet adhesion. Collagen added to platelet-rich patient plasma during aggregation studies mimics this response in vitro and allows for the evaluation of the individual's response to collagen. **Thrombin** activates platelets and protease-activated receptors and induces the complete aggregation of platelets. **Arachidonic acid** elicits granular release and leads to the activation of GpIIb-IIIa. **Adenosine diphosphate** participates in the primary aggregation of platelets by binding to their surface, releasing intracellular calcium, and changing the shape of the platelet.

59. D: Thromboelastography assesses the entire coagulation process based on the properties of clot formation from the start of clot formation, to the maximum stability of a clot, and then to the fibrinolysis-induced resolution of a clot. Whole blood samples are added to a sample cup containing a thin wire that is connected to a mechanical-electrical transducer. As a clot forms in the cup, its elasticity and strength cause the wire to rotate. The rotation is converted to an electrical current that is quantitatively measured and plotted onto a graph. The kinetic, angle, reaction, amplitude, and clot lysis results obtained by thromboelastography aid in the evaluation of the complete clotting process. An **electrochemical** point-of-care test assesses a patient's ability to clot by quantitatively measuring their prothrombin time (PT) and international normalized ratio. Reagent thromboplastin is introduced to patient whole blood samples to initiate the coagulation cascade. Results are obtained by the time elapsed for electrochemical sensors to detect the complete activation of the extrinsic pathway and thrombin conversion. **Bleeding time** evaluations assess capillary function and platelet plug formation by making a small skin incision and drawing off blood from the site every 30 seconds until the bleeding ceases. The time elapsed from when the incision is made to when the bleeding stops is indicative of the platelet number, functionality, adherence to the endothelium, and ability to aggregate. Point-of-care **platelet function assays** measure platelet aggregation in response to specific agonists such as aspirin. Turbidimetric-based assays measure platelet function via optical detection of increased light transmittance emitted by agglutination present in patient samples.

60. B: Nonimmune heparin-induced thrombocytopenia (HIT) and immune HIT are indicated by a decline in platelet counts following heparin therapy. Platelet factor 4 assays detect IgG antibodies and screen patients suspected of HIT. Serotonin release assays confirm an HIT diagnosis by quantifying the amount of serotonin released by platelets in response to reagent HIT antibodies. **Nonimmune HIT** is a direct interaction between heparin and platelets that is classified by platelet counts declining to $\geq 100 \times 10^{12}$/L in the two days following heparin therapy. **Immune HIT** is caused by the development of HIT platelet antibodies and is classified by platelet counts declining to 20–150 × 10^{12}/L at their lowest point five days after the decline begins. Although **lupus anticoagulant** can cause decreased platelet counts, mixing studies are the assays performed to determine its presence. **Protein S activity** is evaluated by performing antigenic C4b-binding protein assays, chromogenic assays, and other functional assays that determine an increased risk of thrombosis.

61. D: Argatroban acts directly on the thrombin enzyme by binding to and blocking its active sites to produce anticoagulant properties. This direct thrombin inhibitor is administered to patients with HIT in efforts to reduce the formation of emboli. The **partial thromboplastin time (PTT)** is the most common coagulation assay performed to monitor the efficacy of direct thrombin inhibitor therapy. The normal reference range for baseline PTT results is 20–40 seconds, with the therapeutic range for argatroban being 1.5–3.0 times greater than the baseline. The **prothrombin time (PT)** assay is performed to monitor warfarin and coumadin therapy, which inhibits the synthesis of vitamin-K-dependent clotting factors. **Thrombin time (TT)** assays monitor fibrinolytic therapy and are greatly affected by the presence of antithrombin agents such as argatroban. **Factor Xa inhibition assays** are performed to monitor the use of medications that directly inhibit factor Xa from converting prothrombin to thrombin.

62. C: Heparin neutralization of a PTT sample occurs due to **introducing heparin** to the sodium citrate tube **during or after a blood draw**. A PTT result can be unexpectedly prolonged if sample tubes are collected in the incorrect order or blood from a tube containing heparin as the anticoagulant is added to a blue sodium citrate tube. In this instance, **intravenous line contamination** is not suspected because there is no heparin running through the line. A **clotting disorder** is not suspected because the patient does not exhibit any symptoms of such a disorder. A prolonged PTT is **not a normal or expected result** in patients without clotting disorders and those who are not receiving heparin therapy and should be investigated.

63. B: Symptoms of **primary** syphilis present at the site of inoculation as a painless lesion, or chancre, 10–90 days following exposure. Primary chancres will resolve on their own in three to six weeks and progress to a secondary infection if untreated. **Secondary** syphilis symptoms include the spread of a diffuse rash that covers the entire body, generalized lymphadenopathy, fatigue, and patchy hair loss that occur 4–12 weeks following the resolution of the primary chancre. Patients with serologic proof of infection who exhibit no signs or symptoms of disease are considered to have **latent** syphilis. Latent infections may return years to decades following the initial infection as late-stage, or **tertiary** syphilis, causing neurological, cardiovascular, and ocular damage that may lead to death.

64. A: The **purified protein derivative (PPD) tuberculin skin test** determines tuberculosis (TB) infection or exposure to *Mycobacterium tuberculosis* by intracutaneously injecting *M. tuberculosis* culture material into the forearm and observing the site 48–72 hours after inoculation. The site of injection is visually inspected for a red, firm bump, known as an induration. The diameter of the induration indicates an individual's tuberculosis status and is interpreted as follows: <5 mm, negative; 5–9 mm, positive for those with HIV, recent contact with someone infected with TB, transplant patients; 10–14 mm, positive for those from areas with a high prevalence of TB, mycobacterial laboratory staff, and children <4 years old; and ≥15mm, positive in all individuals. The **enzyme-linked immunosorbent assay (ELISA)** methodology for diagnosing active and latent TB infections requires whole blood samples to be mixed with synthetic *M. tuberculosis* peptides and incubated. Following incubation, the amount of interferon gamma released by patient lymphocytes is evaluated to determine an individual's TB status, with ≥25% antigenic activity deemed positive for an infection. This ELISA assay is the gold standard for tuberculosis testing and is known as the **interferon gamma release assay** and the **QuantiFERON assay**.

65. B: The bead-based **multiplex immunoassay** is performed by combining a patient sample with cytokine antibody-labeled, color-coded latex beads in a sample well. Cytokines present in the patient sample will bind to their respective antibody-coated bead and remain in the sample well as other biological material is washed away. The beads are separated and detected via flow cytometry, allowing for the qualitative and quantitative measurement of cytokines. Although **ELISA** and **chemiluminescent** methodologies detect cytokines, they are only capable of determining the presence of a single substance at one time. **Rolling cycle amplification** is a molecular methodology and is not used to detect interleukins, growth factors, or interferons.

66. D: Target amplification is an enzyme-mediated technique that detects a target sequence and reproduces the replication process with the use of two oligonucleotide primers. Each individual target amplification method uses this process in unique ways. **Transcription-mediated amplification** methods amplify target nucleic acid sequences in the following manner:

- Primer 1 binds to the target nucleotide.
- Reverse transcriptase initiates polymerization of the strand.
- Reverse transcriptase with RNase H activity degrades the original target strand.
- **Primer 2 binds to the new synthesized strand. Elongation and polymerization form the RNA amplicon, a completed double strand of DNA.**
- RNA polymerase transcribes copies form the amplicon for amplification.

Strand displacement amplification methods target and amplify genetic material with heat denaturation and the following process:

- Two primers concurrently bind to target DNA or RNA. Primer 1 contains a restriction endonuclease and binds to the recognition site of the target strand. Primer 2 attaches next to primer 1.
- **DNA polymerase extends the primers, creating an altered strand that becomes the target for amplification.**
- The new nucleotide target is nicked by restriction endonuclease and displaced to allow the synthesis of more target DNA.

Polymerase chain reaction (PCR) and **ligase chain reaction (LCR)** amplification are completed by repeating the following process in a thermocycler:

- Heat denatures a double-stranded DNA target molecule into two single strands.
- Two primers bind to their complementary nucleotide sequence on the single-stranded DNA templates.
- Elongation occurs by method-specific enzymes:
  - PCR: **DNA polymerase adds nucleotides to the 3′ end of each primer.**
  - LCR: **Taq polymerase adds complementary bases; ligase anneals the appropriate primer to the target DNA probe.**
- Each thermocycle produces double the amount of target DNA.

67. C: Nucleic acid sequence-based amplification methods amplify the genetic material of a target RNA sequence with the use of two genetic primer probes, reverse transcriptase, and RNase H. Molecular beacon probes comprising an oligonucleotide sequence complementary to the target RNA sequence hybridizes to amplified RNA copies and creates a fluorescing strand of DNA. The concentration of target RNA present in a sample is directly proportional to the intensity of the fluorescence emitted by the hybridized sequence. The remaining methods of detection rely on various reactions of molecules but do not obtain information regarding the concentration of genetic material present in the samples. Matrix-assisted laser desorption ionization time-of-flight mass spectrometry (MALDI-TOF MS) separates and detects molecules in a sample, plots the results obtained onto a line graph, and compares the pattern produced to a database of graphs created by known organisms. Pulsed-field gel electrophoresis determines the presence of an organism by forcing a sample through a matrix with electrical currents flowing from various directions. Molecules are detected based on their ability to migrate through the matrix at various distances and create a pattern of bands. Gas chromatography separates samples at the molecular level based on chemical properties, affinity for the column, and the time at which individual molecules elute off of the column.

68. C: Acridine orange is a nonspecific stain that binds to **nucleic acids** of host and bacterial cells. It confirms the presence of bacteria in the following instances: the presence of bacteria is highly suspected, but no bacteria are observed using a light microscope and visualizing bacteria that do not retain Gram stains in their cell wall. **Cellulose and chitin** in the cell wall of fungal elements and parasites fluoresce white on a dark background with calcofluor white stain. **Peptidoglycan layers** in the cell wall of bacteria appear purple or pink when Gram stained and observed with light microscopy. **Mycolic acid** present in the cell wall of mycobacterium appears bright red under a light microscope when acid-fast stained.

69. B: *Streptococcus aureus* resides in the body and on the skin as normal flora, allowing it the most opportunity to become pathogenic in all patients when traumatically introduced to bones and the bloodstream. *Salmonella* species are the most common pathogen responsible for osteomyelitis in patients with sickle cell disease, affecting the long bones in children. Although they can be introduced via traumatic injury, *Brucella* species are most often pathogenic when ingested or inhaled, causing an acute febrile illness that may go undiagnosed and subsequently spread to the bones and surrounding tissue. *Streptococcus agalactiae* causes bone and bloodstream infections in newborns who acquire the infection from the birth canal during labor.

70. C: *Brucella* species organisms have an antigenic lipopolysaccharide outer surface that complement immune complexes cannot easily bind to, allowing the bacteria to evade phagocytosis and proliferate once it enters host cells. O-surface antigens allow *Brucella* to invade host cells, which is necessary for bacterial replication and survival. The ability to survive extreme temperatures and pH levels gives *Brucella* the opportunity to survive in various areas of the body for the establishment and spread of infection. *Salmonella* species possess fimbriae; H, O, and capsular antigens; and antiphagocytic proteins on their surface to aid in the adherence to host cells and prevent phagocytosis and complement-mediated lysis. Lipid A endotoxins released following the death of a *Salmonella* organism are responsible for the fever and shock associated with infections. The peptidoglycan cell wall structure and surface capsular antigens of *Streptococcus aureus* aid in adherence to host cells and preventing phagocytosis, whereas teichoic acids, protein A, and hemolysin and leucocidin toxins contribute to colonization, cell division, and biofilm production associated with infections. The rigid cell wall and polysaccharide capsular antigens of *Streptococcus agalactiae* inhibit the activation of host complement and prevent phagocytosis. The C5a peptidase and pore-forming hemolysins adhere to and gain entry into host cells for replication and survival. The C antigen, cell-surface penicillin-binding protein, and hyaluronidase present on the surface of *S. agalactiae* resist intracellular phagocytosis and promote the spread of infection.

71. A: *Listeria monocytogenes* enters the gastrointestinal tract when contaminated foods such as cheese and vegetables are ingested. Internalin A and B surface proteins on *L. monocytogenes* allow

intracellular access and internalization into gastrointestinal tract epithelial cells. Listeriolysin O and phospholipases aid the bacteria in evading host cell phagocytosis, whereas the actin-assembly-inducing protein generates the force *Listeria* organisms need to become motile and spread from cell to cell within a host. ***Escherichia coli*** can cause neonatal meningitis in newborns exposed to the bacteria in the birth canal during labor. The possession of pili on the surface of *E. coli* aids in their attachment to host cells, with invasin and hemolysin toxins causing disseminated disease.

Neisseria meningitidis and ***Streptococcus pneumoniae*** spread from person to person via respiratory droplets. Both of these organisms have polysaccharide capsular antigens and proteins that allow them to resist phagocytosis and complement-mediated cell lysis.

72. D: ***Clostridium perfringens*** becomes pathogenic when it is introduced into the body by ingesting raw poultry products or from a traumatic injury that introduces the organism via normal skin flora or spores found in soil. The organism invades host cells for survival and proliferation with hemolysins and the following extracellular enzymes: proteases, lipases, collagenase, and hyaluronidase. Alpha, beta, epsilon, and iota toxins produced by varying strains of *C. perfringens* cause damage to surrounding cells, tissues, and blood vessels. *C. perfringens* enterotoxin is secreted following the invasion of intestinal cells and contributes to the virulence of gastrointestinal infections. Infections caused by ***Neisseria*** **species** organisms thrive based on their encapsulation and outer membrane pili that resist phagocytosis and complement-mediated lysis and aid in adherence to host cells. IgA proteases and lipopolysaccharide endotoxins released by *Neisseria* sp. reduce host immune responses by damaging IgA and complement. ***Enterococcus*** organisms possess an intrinsic resistance to beta-lactam and aminoglycoside antibiotics and adhesion factors that induce cell and tissue destruction in hosts, which allow infections to establish and spread to normally sterile sites. **Beta-hemolytic** ***Streptococcus*** **species** invade host cells and encourage the spread of infection with hyaluronidase and evade host immune responses with leukocyte toxic streptolysins S and O. Host immune responses are also suppressed by the *Streptococcal* pyrogenic exotoxin B, which inhibits complement, cytokines, and immunoglobulins.

73. B: Hospital-acquired ***Klebsiella pneumoniae*** infections can occur in immunocompromised patients more than 48 hours after admission by person-to-person contact. *K. pneumoniae* is an encapsulated organism with fimbriae that resist phagocytosis and complement-mediated lysis and enhance adherence to host cells. Lipopolysaccharide endotoxins released by *K. pneumoniae* induce inflammation, and siderophores harvest iron from host cells for the organism's survival. Legionnaires' disease caused by ***Legionella*** is an atypical pneumonia that is acquired by inhaling contaminated water aerosols. The outer membrane of *Legionella* organisms contains a protein that resists phagocytosis. Type IV pili and the release of heat shock protein 60 provides *Legionella* the ability to invade host cells for survival and spread of disease. Tuberculosis infections caused by ***M. tuberculosis*** establish and thrive in the body with the waxy layer and mycolic acid in the organism's cell wall that delay host hypersensitivity and increase antibiotic resistance. Cord factor possessed by *M. tuberculosis* destroys host cell mitochondria and decreases the migration of white blood cells to the site of infection. Toxic lipids and phosphatides released by *M. tuberculosis* also aid in their virulence. ***Mycoplasma pneumoniae*** adheres to host cells in the lungs by evading the body's ciliary clearance response. Community-acquired respiratory distress syndrome toxin allows *M. pneumoniae* to colonize, while causing inflammation and destruction of the airway. Treatment of infections is complicated by the *M. pneumoniae* organism's intrinsic resistance to beta-lactam antibiotics.

74. C: Whooping cough, caused by ***Bordetella pertussis***, most often affects infants who are too young to receive the vaccination. The most common symptoms of the disease are fever, runny nose, nasal congestion, and a severe cough accompanied by a "whoop" sound made during each inhale.

Pertussis is a toxin-mediated disease that establishes and spreads infectious bacteria by way of various antigenic and toxin mechanisms. The filamentous hemagglutinin and pertussis toxins (PTx) 2 and 3 aid in adhesion of bacteria and the colonization required to produce an infection. PTx2 adheres to epithelial cells, whereas PTx3 adheres to phagocytes, inhibiting their phagocytic activity. Once an infection is established, the tracheal cytotoxin released by *B. pertussis* destroys ciliated epithelial cells in the respiratory tract and the lethal toxin causes localized inflammation and tissue necrosis in the lungs and airway. Infections caused by ***Corynebacterium diphtheriae*** present as a fever, sore throat, and swollen lymph nodes in the neck. Diphtheria infections colonize in the respiratory tract with bacterial pili and proteins adhering to various host cells. SpaA, B, and C proteins adhere to epithelial cells in the pharynx, whereas SpaD and H proteins adhere to lung and larynx epithelial cells. *C. diphtheriae* colonization in the respiratory tract forms a thick, gray pseudomembrane that can be observed on the tonsils and in the throat. Spread of the disease is facilitated by the diphtheria toxin, which inhibits protein synthesis in host cells and causes cell death. The toxin is then carried through the bloodstream to other organs where it causes paralysis and congestive heart failure. ***Streptococcus pyogenes*** is the cause of strep throat and pharyngitis, which are characterized by fever, sore throat, painful swallowing, swollen neck lymph nodes, and red, swollen tonsils. Establishment of *S. pyogenes* infections occurs with the hyaluronic acid capsule and M protein preventing phagocytosis and the fibronectin-binding protein and lipoteichoic acids adhering to host epithelial cells. Leukotoxic streptolysins O and S and the streptococcal pyrogenic exotoxin B evade phagocytosis by inhibiting the host immune responses, while spreading factor enzymes invade and destroy connective tissue. ***S. pneumoniae*** causes acute otitis media that can occur along with various other upper respiratory infections such as fever, congestion, headache, and drainage. Infections due to *S. pneumoniae* invade and colonize in hosts by the action of the IgA1 protease and spread by the pore-forming pneumolysin, which lyses host cells that contain cholesterol.

75. A: The **urea breath test** is an indirect, confirmatory method used in the diagnosis of an active *H. pylori* infection and for monitoring the efficacy of treatment in known infections. This method is based on the rapid metabolism of urea and excretion of carbon caused by *H. pylori* infections. Patients ingest urea capsules containing radioactively labeled carbon molecules and exhale into a collection container 10–15 minutes later; then the sample is analyzed for the presence or absence of the labeled carbon molecules. Detection of the labeled molecules confirms the diagnosis of a new *H. pylori* infection or determines that an infection undergoing antibiotic treatment has not yet been eradicated. The detection of *H. pylori* antigens with **serological IgG antibodies** is also an indirect method. However, antigen detection via monoclonal or polyclonal *H. pylori* antibodies does not differentiate between past or presently active infections and requires the performance of a second method of testing to confirm an active infection. **PCR** and **rapid urease testing methods** directly detect the presence of *H. pylori* organisms. PCR testing targets an organism-specific sequence of DNA and amplifies the sequence for detection and identification of an infection. The rapid urease testing method confirms an active *H. pylori* infection in 1–24 hours with the addition of an intestinal biopsy specimen to agar or a test strip containing urea, a buffer, and pH indicator. The presence of an active *H. pylori* infection is confirmed by an alkaline change in the pH due to ammonia production.

76. B: ***Bacteroides fragilis*** is a commensal organism in the intestines, but it becomes pathogenic when it is displaced into other soft tissues or near bone. Due to its encapsulation, *B. fragilis* resists phagocytosis by host cells and induces the formation of abscesses. Beta-lactamase production renders beta-lactam antibiotics ineffective for treating *B. fragilis* infections. ***Pseudomonas aeruginosa*** also evades phagocytosis and complement-mediated lysis via encapsulation, but it is an aerobic organism that resides as normal flora on the skin and in the intestines. Additional virulence mechanisms of *P. aeruginosa* include proteases that decrease the effectiveness of host IgA and complement and the exotoxin A that is toxic to macrophages. Although *P. mirabilis* is also part of the intestinal normal flora, this organism is not encapsulated. *Proteus mirabilis* has flagella and outer-membrane antigens that aid in its virulence, as well as fimbriae that allow for adhesion to host cells. *Prevotella* **species'** mechanisms for establishing an infection include adhering to the surface of host cells, while producing proteases to damage host IgA and complement and hemolysins that lyse host red blood cells.

77. C: Infections caused by *Mycoplasma* species can be diagnosed by culture and molecular methods. Molecular testing has become the method of choice due to its high sensitivity and time efficiency. PCR and nucleic acid amplification testing (NAAT) methods allow for the rapid diagnosis of genital tract infections caused by *Mycoplasma* by targeting and amplifying a specific gene of nucleic acid sequence. *Mycoplasma genitalium* is a common cause of sexually transmitted infections (STIs) and requires differentiation from other STI pathogens such as *C. trachomatis* and *Neisseria gonorrhoeae*. **NAAT methods** allow for the rapid diagnosis of *M. genitalium* infections based on the amplification and detection of the species-specific ***tuf* gene. Fluorochrome acridine orange stain** confirms the presence of bacteria that cannot be observed via light microscopy or does not retain the Gram stain, including *Mycoplasma* organisms. The nonspecific stain binds to nucleic acids of bacteria and host cells and produces a bright-orange color on a dark background. Although the acridine orange stain can detect the presence of bacteria, this method cannot differentiate organisms or diagnose the cause of an infection. Although detecting *Mycoplasma* on culture media is highly specific to the bacteria and confirms an infection, this method is time consuming, has specific growth requirements, and requires expertly trained staff. *Mycoplasma* **colonies appear small and inverted, resembling a fried egg, following four weeks of incubation** under the following conditions: **sterol-enriched media incubated at 35–37 °C in a 95% nitrogen and 5% carbon dioxide** environment. All species of *Mycoplasma* appear the same on culture media, which does not allow for the differentiation and species-specific identification that molecular methods achieve.

78. A: Infections caused by each of these organisms can be sexually transmitted and cause symptoms of the genital tract. *N. gonorrhoeae*, *Gardnerella vaginalis*, and *C. trachomatis* demonstrate similar symptoms of painful urination, vaginal and penile discharge, pain, and irritation. However, each of these organisms has species-specific virulence mechanisms and methods of establishing an infection. *N. gonorrhoeae* possesses pili with antiphagocytic properties to aid in the adherence to host mucosal cells and IgA protease that hydrolyzes host IgA-mediated immune responses and allows for the establishment of an infection. *C. trachomatis* exists in two forms: the infectious, extracellular elementary body and the noninfectious, intracellular reticulate body. The elementary body of *C. trachomatis* contains outer membrane proteins for adherence and entrance into host cells, whereas the reticulate body replicates intracellularly and possesses chlamydial proteasome, which degrades host cell DNA. The virulence of *G. vaginalis* is based on the activity of vaginolysin, which adheres to and is cytotoxic to host cells, and sialidase, which promotes colonization and the formation of a biofilm. *T. pallidum* infections are characterized by a small, painless sore known as a chancre that occurs at the site of inoculation. The chancre may go unnoticed and resolve on its own, leading to secondary syphilis symptoms to occurs weeks later as a systemic skin rash. *T. pallidum* contains fibronectin, which decreases the phagocytic properties of macrophages; outer membrane proteins, which aid in adherence; and hyaluronidase, which allows infiltration into host cells.

79. A: 16s rRNA gene sequencing is a methodology that allows for the identification and classification of bacteria in complex biological mixtures, including the gastrointestinal microbiome. Sequencing uses probes to detect and amplify multiple variable regions on the bacterial 16s ribosomal gene that provides information for the further classification of organisms. The phylogenetic nature of this method detects variable regions specific to the expression of *C. diff* toxins A and B, which aid in the diagnosis of an active *C. diff* infection in symptomatic patients. **PCR methods** are often used in conjunction with 16s rRNA sequencing to effectively amplify and detect specific toxigenic genes in a time-efficient manner. Stand-alone PCR methodologies with primer probes are also available; however, they do not use the same mechanisms as gene sequencing methods. Commercial **enzyme immunoassay (EIA)** test kits for the detection of toxigenic *C. diff* are available for the rapid detection of an infection. Enzyme immunoassay tests are embedded with monoclonal antibodies that will combine with **C. diff toxin** and **glutamate dehydrogenase (GDH) antigens** if they are present in a sample. The antigen–antibody complex formed will react with a substrate to produce a visible colored line in the test kit. *C. diff* toxin and GDH antibodies are embedded in separate portions of the test window to differentiate their presence. The absence of a line for the toxin and the GDH antigen accurately rules out *C. diff* as a cause for infection. However, the presence of a line for one or both of these requires further workup and correlation with clinical signs and symptoms.

80. D: Glycopeptide antibiotics are bactericidal agents for Gram-positive bacteria and the drug of choice for methicillin-resistant *Staphylococcus aureus* and *C. diff* infections. This class of drugs binds to peptidoglycan precursors in the cell wall of bacteria, inhibiting cell wall synthesis and causing cell lysis. Bactericidal **aminoglycoside** antibiotics act against Gram-negative organisms by binding to bacterial RNA in the ribosomes, inhibiting protein synthesis, and causing cell death. **Beta-lactam** antibiotics cause cell death in Gram-positive and Gram-negative organisms by binding to the penicillin-binding protein and inactivating cell wall synthesis. **Macrolides** are bacteriostatic agents that inhibit protein-binding synthesis of Gram-positive organisms, which prevents bacterial growth and multiplication.

81. B: Hospital inpatients are often screened for the presence of antibiotic-resistant bacteria in their nasal passages or gastrointestinal tract upon admission. Early detection of antibiotic-resistant organisms allows for more insight into potential sources of infection and treatment options, as well as the implementation of appropriate infection control measures to protect patients and staff against the spread of potential pathogens. Rectal or perianal swabs are collected to screen for gastrointestinal colonization of vancomycin-resistant *Enterococci*, carbapenemase-resistant *Enterobacteriaceae*, and extended-spectrum beta-lactamase organisms. Methicillin-resistant *S. aureus* colonization of the mucous membrane is screened for by swabbing just inside each nostril. Molecular methods are used to detect specific genes that are known to express antimicrobial resistance and require alternative courses of treatment if opportunistic organisms become pathogenic. PCR methods detect antimicrobial-resistant bacteria with gene-specific primers and probes. Detection of the following genes indicates colonization of their respective antibiotic-resistant organisms:

- **vanA:** vancomycin-resistant *Enterococci*
- **Beta-lactamase:** extended-spectrum beta-lactamase organisms
- **Carbapenemase:** carbapenem-resistant *Enterobacteriaceae*
- **mecA:** methicillin-resistant *S. aureus*

82. D: Each of the organisms listed is categorized as a biosafety level three (BSL-3) pathogen based on their highly infectious nature and ability to cause disease following the inhalation of contaminated aerosols. BSL-3 agents require the use of a biological safety hood in the laboratory to reduce the potential of transmission to staff members who are cultivating and analyzing the organisms. Aerosol inhalation of each of these organisms has the potential to cause serious and highly contagious pneumonic diseases in humans.

Francisella tularensis is a zoonotic disease that affects humans following the inhalation of the organism in landscaping, farming, and laboratory settings. The pneumonic form of the disease presents as a fever, cough, chest pain, and difficulty breathing. Tularemia can also present as infections of the skin, glands, throat, or eyes based on its point of entry into the body. *M. tuberculosis* infections occur due to the inhalation of contaminated respiratory droplets and present with the following symptoms: a cough lasting three or more weeks, chest pain, fever, chills, night sweats, fatigue, and bloody sputum. *Yersinia pestis* can be transmitted to humans via infected tick bites or from person to person by inhaling contaminated aerosols. Pneumonic infections of the plague cause fever, headache, weakness, shortness of breath, chest pain, and bloody or watery mucus in those affected. *Bacillus anthracis* occurs naturally in soil, infects various domestic and wild animals, and enters the human body via inhalation of spores, ingestion of contaminated food or water, and through traumatic inoculation in the skin. Pneumonic anthrax infections present with the following symptoms: fever and chills, chest pain, shortness of breath, confusion and dizziness, extreme fatigue, nausea and vomiting, cough, and body aches.

F. tularensis, *B. anthracis*, and *Y. pestis* organisms are all encapsulated with a lipopolysaccharide outer membrane that aids in the invasion into host cells and prevents phagocytosis by host defenses. The cell wall of *M. tuberculosis* also defeats host and antibiotic defenses with a waxy mycolic layer. *F. tularensis* and *Y. pestis* contain pili that allow the bacteria to adhere to and invade host cells, which is pertinent to bacterial survival in hosts. Additionally, *F. tularensis* prevents phagocytosis with the action of acid phosphatase and sequesters iron from host cells with siderosomes. Plasminogen activators and fibrinolysin produced by *Y. pestis* are cytotoxic to host cells and prevent phagosome opsonization, which aid in the spread of disease. A combination of three exotoxins produced by *B. anthracis* allows the organism to bind to, enter, and destroy host cells for the establishment and spread of the infection. The three exotoxins, protective antigen, edema factor, and lethal factor, combine to form this anthrax toxin. *M. tuberculosis* decreases host defenses with lipoarabinomannan and the ESX 1 secretory system. Lipoarabinomannan aids in adhesion and prevents interferon-mediated action, cytokine production and release, and T lymphocyte proliferation in infected people. The ESX 1 secretory system prevents host phagocytosis by decreasing phagosome-lysosome fusion.

83. C: Matrix-assisted laser desorption ionization time-of-flight mass spectrometry (MALDI-TOF MS) is a two-phase process that identifies organisms by separating and detecting them on a molecular level. The first phase of the process involves the fixation of a suspension containing a bacterial colony to a crystalline matrix. The matrix is blasted by a laser, which vaporizes the suspension, ionizing the molecules without fragmenting or destroying them. TOF MS is the second phase of the process in which molecules are separated based on their mass-to-charge ratio, and they are then measured by the time it takes for each molecule to travel to the detector. The data produced by this process are plotted onto a line graph and compared to a catalog with graphs of known organisms. MALDI-TOF MS allows for differentiation and identification of organisms with similar reactions to biochemical tests and antimicrobials. *Mycobacteria* and *Nocardia* species can be differentiated from one another, and each genus can be identified to the species level. **NAAT, restriction endonuclease amplification,** and **16s ribosomal RNA sequencing** are also molecular methods used in the detection of the *Mycobacteria* and *Nocardia* species of pathogens. **NAAT** methods detect specific organisms in the following manner:

- Ribosomal RNA is targeted and amplified.
- The target sequence anneals to the primer probes and amplifies.
- Amplified sequences are attached to chemiluminescent labeled probes for detection.

Restriction endonuclease amplification detects *Nocardia* species-specific proteins and genes in the following manner:

- Primer 1, containing a restriction endonuclease, attaches at the recognition site of the target DNA or RNA sequence.
- Primer 2 attaches to the target strand adjacent to primer 1.
- Polymerase extends the primer, creating an altered strand that becomes the new target for amplification.
- The new target strand is nicked by restriction endonuclease and displaces the strand.
- Primers attach to the new strand, and the process repeats, amplifying the target sequences.

The **16s ribosomal gene sequencing** method uses primer tools to amplify variable regions on the 16s-ribosomal gene in the bacterial genome. Variable regions V2, V3, V4, V6, V7, V8, and V9 on the gene are targeted to produce a genetic sequence unique to each species of bacteria. Sequences derived from genetic sequencing are compared to a database containing reference sequences for organisms, allowing for species-specific identification.

84. A: Treatment of an active *M. tuberculosis* infection is a multifaceted process that requires the use of multiple classes of antibiotics over an extended period of time. Isoniazid, rifampin, and ethambutol administered over a length of 6–18 months are commonly prescribed to eradicate the infection. The beta subunit of the **RNA polymerase gene** mediates the resistance to rifampin, whereas the **catalase gene** mediates the resistance to isoniazid. Nucleic acid amplification techniques are available to detect the expression of these genes and provide further insight on the most appropriate treatment for an *M. tuberculosis* infection. Gene sequencing and PCR methods are combined to detect **gyrase B** and **65-kDa heat shock protein genes** for the differentiation of *Nocardia* species organisms that are biochemically indistinguishable.

85. B: *Mycobacteria* and *Nocardia* infections require treatment with multiple antibiotics over extended periods of time due to their high incidence of antimicrobial resistance. Infections caused by **nontuberculous *Mycobacteria*** are treated with a combination of rifampin and ethambutol antibiotics over the course of 6–12 months. *M. tuberculosis* infections are treated for a minimum of 6 months up to 18 months with a macrolide, followed by a combination of rifampin and ethambutol antimicrobials. **Localized *Nocardia*** infections are eradicated with sulfonamide drugs, with treatment lasting 6–12 months depending on the severity. **Systemic nocardiosis** requires 6–12 months of treatment with a combination of a sulfonamide and amikacin or one of the other following primary agents: ceftriaxone, cefotaxime, linezolid, or imipenem.

86. C: *Nocardia* **species** organisms naturally reside in the soil and water and participate in the decomposition of plant material. These organisms become pathogenic when they are inhaled or enter the skin via traumatic inoculation. Skin abscesses form during *Nocardia* infections due to the organism's ability to deter the host immune system with the following virulence mechanisms: inhibiting phagosome-lysosome fusion during phagocytosis, resisting the antimicrobial action of neutrophils, and causing cell death with catalase and hemolysin, respectively. **Nontuberculous *Mycobacteria*** also occurs naturally in the environment; however, most infections are caused by the insertion of prosthetic devices and the establishment of infection relies on adherence to host cells and the formation of a biofilm. *S. aureus* and *S. pyogenes* are both part of the normal skin flora that become pathogenic and capable of forming an abscess when they enter the body through a break in the skin. *S. aureus'* rigid cell wall and capsular antigens evade phagocytosis and promote adherence to host cells. Adhesion, colonization, and spread of an *S. aureus* infection is made possible by teichoic acids, protein A, hemolysins, leucocidin, and various enzymes. *S. pyogenes* can cause erysipelas, a superficial cutaneous infection of the face or legs. A hyaluronic acid capsule prevents the phagocytosis of *S. pyogenes*, whereas the fibronectin-binding protein, M protein, and lipoteichoic acids aid in adhesion to host cells and streptolysins S and O destroy host leukocytes.

87. C: The large intestinal roundworm *Ascaris lumbricoides* can be detected macroscopically in stool samples by adult worms that measure six inches to over a foot long. Adult female worms are typically longer than adult males and have a straight tail compared to the males' curved tail. Adult tapeworm proglottids of *Taenia solium,* the pork tapeworm, macroscopically detected in stool samples are flat, ribbon-like, segmented worms. The broad fish tapeworm, *Diphyllobothrium latum,* can also be detected by macroscopically observing adult proglottid tapeworms that can be inches to several feet long. *Enterobius vermicularis* is most commonly identified by the presence of larvae around the perianal area. Cellulose tape is pressed up against the area, and any pinworm eggs or larva present will be collected for microscopic evaluation. Pinworm larvae can be visualized moving outside the anus by shining a flashlight at the perianal area. Adult pinworms can get stuck to the outside of stool samples when they pass through the anus.

88. A: *Cryptococcus neoformans* appears as white or cream-colored smooth mucoid colonies after 48–72 hours of incubation at 37 °C in 5% CO_2 on Sabouraud dextrose agar (SDA). *Histoplasma capsulatum* grows on SDA at 25–37 °C, with colonies appearing white and fluffy within five days of incubation and turning a buff to brown color as they age. Following 24–48 hours of incubation at 25–37 °C, *Candida albicans* grows into cream-colored smooth colonies with a yeast-like odor. *Aspergillus fumigatus* colonies appear blue-green and velvety with a narrow white margin on the front of SDA and a pale-yellow color on the back of the media following 72 hours of incubation at 25–45 °C.

89. D: Wright's stain is a hematologic stain that allows for the differentiation of blood cells under light microscopy. Bone marrow, peripheral blood smears, and urine samples are most suitable for staining with Wright's stain. *H. capsulatum*, an intracellular yeast that appears in mononuclear and epithelial cells, appear following Wright's stain as round to oval cells that measure 2–5 μm in diameter. The **acid-fast** stain is performed to determine the presence of organisms whose cell walls contain mycolic acid and do not retain the Gram stain. Acid-fast *Mycobacteria* and partial acid-fast *Nocardia* are detected via this stain, appearing bright red and pink, respectively. Yeast and fungi do not contain mycolic acid in the cell wall and appear as blue with the counterstain. **Calcofluor white** stain is often used in conjunction with potassium hydroxide (KOH) reagent to visualize all fungal elements. KOH breaks down the keratin present in hair and nail samples and clears excess debris to allow for fungal elements to be more easily observed. Fungal elements stained with calcofluor white fluoresce bright green, whereas other organisms appear bright red on a dark field. Despite the cell wall containing cellulose and chitin, *H. capsulatum* often stains poorly with the nonspecific calcofluor white stain. **India ink** is a diagnostic stain for *C. neoformans*, which appears on a dark field as spherical, single- or multibudding yeast, 2–15 μm in diameter, with a thick wall and a wide retractile capsule.

90. B: The **urease test** allows for rapid determination between the common pathogen *C. albicans* that is urease negative and the potentially fatal *C. neoformans* that is urease positive. Organisms that produce urease hydrolyze urea, which releases ammonia and causes an alkaline shift in pH.

The process of the test uses pH paper with a phenol color indicator to determine the production of urease. A bacterial colony suspended in saline is placed on the pH paper, and a color change from yellow to magenta confirms this biochemical change. The **germ tube test** is a direct method used to differentiate *C. albicans* from other *Candida* species organisms. The process is based on the ability of *C. albicans* to produce germ tubes, or hypha-like extensions with no constrictions, from its yeast cells. *C. neoformans* cannot be identified or excluded as a potential pathogen using this method. Serological methods can be used for the rapid identification of *C. neoformans*. The *C. neoformans* **capsular antigen** present during infection will bind to antibody-coated latex beads and form a visible agglutinate. However, these methods require serum or cerebrospinal fluid samples and cannot be completed using a culture colony. Direct detection and differentiation of *C. neoformans* and *C. albicans* can be made by observing an isolate that has been stained with **India ink**. *C. neoformans* presents as an encapsulated yeast with no pseudohyphae, whereas *C. albicans* appears as small, extracellular yeast with pseudohyphae. Although the capsular antigen latex agglutination and India ink methods are able to rapidly detect *C. neoformans*, they are not based on biochemical reactions.

91. D: The **gas chromatography-mass spectrometry** methodology is the "gold standard" for confirming the presence and concentration of drugs and drug metabolites. The combination of separation and detection processes allows for a highly sensitive and reliable method. Gas chromatography separates molecules in a sample based on their unique chemical properties and affinity for the capillary column, which determines the speed that they elute from the column and into the mass spectrometer. Mass spectrometry fragments large molecules and subtracts electrons from small molecules for ionization and focuses ionized molecules into a beam. The beam increases the kinetic energy of each ionized molecule and allows them to pass through a magnetic field. In the magnetic field, molecular **ions are deflected into the detector at varying speeds and directions** based on their mass-to-charge ratio. Data produced from the detector are plotted on a line graph and compared to graphs of known substances and compounds. **Spectrophotometric** methods determine the concentration of a substance in a sample based on the **production of color.** Analytes are quantitively measured by comparing the color produced by a reaction to the color observed at known concentrations. Although spectrophotometry is used to measure various analytes, it is not a method that is used to confirm the presence of drugs. Thin-layer chromatography and immunoassay methods are used to screen for the presence or absence of drugs and require repeat analysis by a second, confirmatory method. **Thin-layer chromatography** detects various substances in a sample based on the **distance and pattern of their migration** through a thin layer of adsorbent material. **Immunoassay** methodologies are based on the reaction between **monoclonal antibodies** for each drug class and drug metabolites or a chromatic conjugate. When a drug is not present, the antibody will bind to the conjugate and migrate to the test line for the specific drug class, producing a colored line. A drug present in the sample will bind to antibodies embedded in the test cartridge instead of the conjugate, and no color is produced.

92. C: Professional ethics are a set of principles that determine the proper conduct for an individual or group to follow in the workplace. **Personal ethics** are principles established by each individual that help them navigate decision making and other situations. **Medical** ethics are established principles that are specific to resolution and proper conduct in a clinical setting. **Beneficence** is a single principle that is included in professional and medical ethics established for healthcare workers, which states that healthcare professionals must do all they can to benefit the patient in each healthcare situation that they are a part of.

93. A: Under HIPAA, a patient's protected health information may be shared with family members or other designated individuals only after the patient has consented and the proper documentation has been made. Results and patient demographics for reportable diseases are able to be shared with public health departments without prior patient consent. Demographics are provided to public health departments to record and track communicable diseases within an area and contact others affected if necessary. Laboratory staff are able to access laboratory results of their family members only when it is necessary for a job-related task. Accessing results under any other circumstances is deemed a violation of HIPAA. When the validation of current laboratory results or correlation with prior results is required, accessing prior diagnoses or laboratory results is allowed under HIPAA.

94. C: The integration of result autoverification into laboratory processes reduces the need for staff to manually review and verify every result, effectively increasing productivity and efficiency. The **postanalytical phase** of the laboratory process occurs after specimen processing has been completed and entails the following actions: result transmission and interpretation, critical value retesting and reporting, and evaluation of laboratory statistical data. Laboratory information systems (LIS) aid in **preanalytical** processes by automatically linking a patient's information with previous encounters, through their medical record number, and providing unique identifiers for each encounter to ensure that tests and results are entered for the appropriate visit. LIS-generated bar codes are also an advantage of automation during the preanalytical phase by assisting with proper patient identification, sample collection, and storage. Once testing and the **analytical** phase begin, LIS-generated bar codes link samples on the analyzer to their corresponding test requisitions and implement the assays requested for each individual patient sample.

95. B: Although the technologist determines that the A1C calibration is expired after the patient has been processed, this error falls into the analytical phase of the laboratory process. Assuring the validity method of calibrations is part of analyzer and analyte maintenance and is deemed an analytical task. Issues regarding sample collection and reagent storage occur prior to the analysis of a sample and are examples of preanalytical errors. Clerical errors can be made during the pre- and postanalytical phases of laboratory processes. The release of patient results under the wrong patient requisition is a postanalytical error because it was made after testing had been completed.

How to Overcome Test Anxiety

Just the thought of taking a test is enough to make most people a little nervous. A test is an important event that can have a long-term impact on your future, so it's important to take it seriously and it's natural to feel anxious about performing well. But just because anxiety is normal, that doesn't mean that it's helpful in test taking, or that you should simply accept it as part of your life. Anxiety can have a variety of effects. These effects can be mild, like making you feel slightly nervous, or severe, like blocking your ability to focus or remember even a simple detail.

If you experience test anxiety—whether severe or mild—it's important to know how to beat it. To discover this, first you need to understand what causes test anxiety.

Causes of Test Anxiety

While we often think of anxiety as an uncontrollable emotional state, it can actually be caused by simple, practical things. One of the most common causes of test anxiety is that a person does not feel adequately prepared for their test. This feeling can be the result of many different issues such as poor study habits or lack of organization, but the most common culprit is time management. Starting to study too late, failing to organize your study time to cover all of the material, or being distracted while you study will mean that you're not well prepared for the test. This may lead to cramming the night before, which will cause you to be physically and mentally exhausted for the test. Poor time management also contributes to feelings of stress, fear, and hopelessness as you realize you are not well prepared but don't know what to do about it.

Other times, test anxiety is not related to your preparation for the test but comes from unresolved fear. This may be a past failure on a test, or poor performance on tests in general. It may come from comparing yourself to others who seem to be performing better or from the stress of living up to expectations. Anxiety may be driven by fears of the future—how failure on this test would affect your educational and career goals. These fears are often completely irrational, but they can still negatively impact your test performance.

> **Review Video:** <u>3 Reasons You Have Test Anxiety</u>
> Visit mometrix.com/academy and enter code: 428468

Elements of Test Anxiety

As mentioned earlier, test anxiety is considered to be an emotional state, but it has physical and mental components as well. Sometimes you may not even realize that you are suffering from test anxiety until you notice the physical symptoms. These can include trembling hands, rapid heartbeat, sweating, nausea, and tense muscles. Extreme anxiety may lead to fainting or vomiting. Obviously, any of these symptoms can have a negative impact on testing. It is important to recognize them as soon as they begin to occur so that you can address the problem before it damages your performance.

> **Review Video: 3 Ways to Tell You Have Test Anxiety**
> Visit mometrix.com/academy and enter code: 927847

The mental components of test anxiety include trouble focusing and inability to remember learned information. During a test, your mind is on high alert, which can help you recall information and stay focused for an extended period of time. However, anxiety interferes with your mind's natural processes, causing you to blank out, even on the questions you know well. The strain of testing during anxiety makes it difficult to stay focused, especially on a test that may take several hours. Extreme anxiety can take a huge mental toll, making it difficult not only to recall test information but even to understand the test questions or pull your thoughts together.

> **Review Video: How Test Anxiety Affects Memory**
> Visit mometrix.com/academy and enter code: 609003

Effects of Test Anxiety

Test anxiety is like a disease—if left untreated, it will get progressively worse. Anxiety leads to poor performance, and this reinforces the feelings of fear and failure, which in turn lead to poor performances on subsequent tests. It can grow from a mild nervousness to a crippling condition. If allowed to progress, test anxiety can have a big impact on your schooling, and consequently on your future.

Test anxiety can spread to other parts of your life. Anxiety on tests can become anxiety in any stressful situation, and blanking on a test can turn into panicking in a job situation. But fortunately, you don't have to let anxiety rule your testing and determine your grades. There are a number of relatively simple steps you can take to move past anxiety and function normally on a test and in the rest of life.

> **Review Video: How Test Anxiety Impacts Your Grades**
> Visit mometrix.com/academy and enter code: 939819

Physical Steps for Beating Test Anxiety

While test anxiety is a serious problem, the good news is that it can be overcome. It doesn't have to control your ability to think and remember information. While it may take time, you can begin taking steps today to beat anxiety.

Just as your first hint that you may be struggling with anxiety comes from the physical symptoms, the first step to treating it is also physical. Rest is crucial for having a clear, strong mind. If you are tired, it is much easier to give in to anxiety. But if you establish good sleep habits, your body and mind will be ready to perform optimally, without the strain of exhaustion. Additionally, sleeping well helps you to retain information better, so you're more likely to recall the answers when you see the test questions.

Getting good sleep means more than going to bed on time. It's important to allow your brain time to relax. Take study breaks from time to time so it doesn't get overworked, and don't study right before bed. Take time to rest your mind before trying to rest your body, or you may find it difficult to fall asleep.

> **Review Video: <u>The Importance of Sleep for Your Brain</u>**
> Visit mometrix.com/academy and enter code: 319338

Along with sleep, other aspects of physical health are important in preparing for a test. Good nutrition is vital for good brain function. Sugary foods and drinks may give a burst of energy but this burst is followed by a crash, both physically and emotionally. Instead, fuel your body with protein and vitamin-rich foods.

Also, drink plenty of water. Dehydration can lead to headaches and exhaustion, especially if your brain is already under stress from the rigors of the test. Particularly if your test is a long one, drink water during the breaks. And if possible, take an energy-boosting snack to eat between sections.

> **Review Video: <u>How Diet Can Affect your Mood</u>**
> Visit mometrix.com/academy and enter code: 624317

Along with sleep and diet, a third important part of physical health is exercise. Maintaining a steady workout schedule is helpful, but even taking 5-minute study breaks to walk can help get your blood pumping faster and clear your head. Exercise also releases endorphins, which contribute to a positive feeling and can help combat test anxiety.

When you nurture your physical health, you are also contributing to your mental health. If your body is healthy, your mind is much more likely to be healthy as well. So take time to rest, nourish your body with healthy food and water, and get moving as much as possible. Taking these physical steps will make you stronger and more able to take the mental steps necessary to overcome test anxiety.

Mental Steps for Beating Test Anxiety

Working on the mental side of test anxiety can be more challenging, but as with the physical side, there are clear steps you can take to overcome it. As mentioned earlier, test anxiety often stems from lack of preparation, so the obvious solution is to prepare for the test. Effective studying may be the most important weapon you have for beating test anxiety, but you can and should employ several other mental tools to combat fear.

First, boost your confidence by reminding yourself of past success—tests or projects that you aced. If you're putting as much effort into preparing for this test as you did for those, there's no reason you should expect to fail here. Work hard to prepare; then trust your preparation.

Second, surround yourself with encouraging people. It can be helpful to find a study group, but be sure that the people you're around will encourage a positive attitude. If you spend time with others who are anxious or cynical, this will only contribute to your own anxiety. Look for others who are motivated to study hard from a desire to succeed, not from a fear of failure.

Third, reward yourself. A test is physically and mentally tiring, even without anxiety, and it can be helpful to have something to look forward to. Plan an activity following the test, regardless of the outcome, such as going to a movie or getting ice cream.

When you are taking the test, if you find yourself beginning to feel anxious, remind yourself that you know the material. Visualize successfully completing the test. Then take a few deep, relaxing breaths and return to it. Work through the questions carefully but with confidence, knowing that you are capable of succeeding.

Developing a healthy mental approach to test taking will also aid in other areas of life. Test anxiety affects more than just the actual test—it can be damaging to your mental health and even contribute to depression. It's important to beat test anxiety before it becomes a problem for more than testing.

> **Review Video: Test Anxiety and Depression**
> Visit mometrix.com/academy and enter code: 904704

Study Strategy

Being prepared for the test is necessary to combat anxiety, but what does being prepared look like? You may study for hours on end and still not feel prepared. What you need is a strategy for test prep. The next few pages outline our recommended steps to help you plan out and conquer the challenge of preparation.

STEP 1: SCOPE OUT THE TEST

Learn everything you can about the format (multiple choice, essay, etc.) and what will be on the test. Gather any study materials, course outlines, or sample exams that may be available. Not only will this help you to prepare, but knowing what to expect can help to alleviate test anxiety.

STEP 2: MAP OUT THE MATERIAL

Look through the textbook or study guide and make note of how many chapters or sections it has. Then divide these over the time you have. For example, if a book has 15 chapters and you have five days to study, you need to cover three chapters each day. Even better, if you have the time, leave an extra day at the end for overall review after you have gone through the material in depth.

If time is limited, you may need to prioritize the material. Look through it and make note of which sections you think you already have a good grasp on, and which need review. While you are studying, skim quickly through the familiar sections and take more time on the challenging parts. Write out your plan so you don't get lost as you go. Having a written plan also helps you feel more in control of the study, so anxiety is less likely to arise from feeling overwhelmed at the amount to cover.

STEP 3: GATHER YOUR TOOLS

Decide what study method works best for you. Do you prefer to highlight in the book as you study and then go back over the highlighted portions? Or do you type out notes of the important information? Or is it helpful to make flashcards that you can carry with you? Assemble the pens, index cards, highlighters, post-it notes, and any other materials you may need so you won't be distracted by getting up to find things while you study.

If you're having a hard time retaining the information or organizing your notes, experiment with different methods. For example, try color-coding by subject with colored pens, highlighters, or post-it notes. If you learn better by hearing, try recording yourself reading your notes so you can listen while in the car, working out, or simply sitting at your desk. Ask a friend to quiz you from your flashcards, or try teaching someone the material to solidify it in your mind.

STEP 4: CREATE YOUR ENVIRONMENT

It's important to avoid distractions while you study. This includes both the obvious distractions like visitors and the subtle distractions like an uncomfortable chair (or a too-comfortable couch that makes you want to fall asleep). Set up the best study environment possible: good lighting and a comfortable work area. If background music helps you focus, you may want to turn it on, but otherwise keep the room quiet. If you are using a computer to take notes, be sure you don't have any other windows open, especially applications like social media, games, or anything else that could distract you. Silence your phone and turn off notifications. Be sure to keep water close by so you stay hydrated while you study (but avoid unhealthy drinks and snacks).

Also, take into account the best time of day to study. Are you freshest first thing in the morning? Try to set aside some time then to work through the material. Is your mind clearer in the afternoon or evening? Schedule your study session then. Another method is to study at the same time of day that you will take the test, so that your brain gets used to working on the material at that time and will be ready to focus at test time.

STEP 5: STUDY!

Once you have done all the study preparation, it's time to settle into the actual studying. Sit down, take a few moments to settle your mind so you can focus, and begin to follow your study plan. Don't give in to distractions or let yourself procrastinate. This is your time to prepare so you'll be ready to fearlessly approach the test. Make the most of the time and stay focused.

Of course, you don't want to burn out. If you study too long you may find that you're not retaining the information very well. Take regular study breaks. For example, taking five minutes out of every hour to walk briskly, breathing deeply and swinging your arms, can help your mind stay fresh.

As you get to the end of each chapter or section, it's a good idea to do a quick review. Remind yourself of what you learned and work on any difficult parts. When you feel that you've mastered the material, move on to the next part. At the end of your study session, briefly skim through your notes again.

But while review is helpful, cramming last minute is NOT. If at all possible, work ahead so that you won't need to fit all your study into the last day. Cramming overloads your brain with more information than it can process and retain, and your tired mind may struggle to recall even previously learned information when it is overwhelmed with last-minute study. Also, the urgent nature of cramming and the stress placed on your brain contribute to anxiety. You'll be more likely to go to the test feeling unprepared and having trouble thinking clearly.

So don't cram, and don't stay up late before the test, even just to review your notes at a leisurely pace. Your brain needs rest more than it needs to go over the information again. In fact, plan to finish your studies by noon or early afternoon the day before the test. Give your brain the rest of the day to relax or focus on other things, and get a good night's sleep. Then you will be fresh for the test and better able to recall what you've studied.

STEP 6: TAKE A PRACTICE TEST

Many courses offer sample tests, either online or in the study materials. This is an excellent resource to check whether you have mastered the material, as well as to prepare for the test format and environment.

Check the test format ahead of time: the number of questions, the type (multiple choice, free response, etc.), and the time limit. Then create a plan for working through them. For example, if you have 30 minutes to take a 60-question test, your limit is 30 seconds per question. Spend less time on the questions you know well so that you can take more time on the difficult ones.

If you have time to take several practice tests, take the first one open book, with no time limit. Work through the questions at your own pace and make sure you fully understand them. Gradually work up to taking a test under test conditions: sit at a desk with all study materials put away and set a timer. Pace yourself to make sure you finish the test with time to spare and go back to check your answers if you have time.

After each test, check your answers. On the questions you missed, be sure you understand why you missed them. Did you misread the question (tests can use tricky wording)? Did you forget the information? Or was it something you hadn't learned? Go back and study any shaky areas that the practice tests reveal.

141

Taking these tests not only helps with your grade, but also aids in combating test anxiety. If you're already used to the test conditions, you're less likely to worry about it, and working through tests until you're scoring well gives you a confidence boost. Go through the practice tests until you feel comfortable, and then you can go into the test knowing that you're ready for it.

Test Tips

On test day, you should be confident, knowing that you've prepared well and are ready to answer the questions. But aside from preparation, there are several test day strategies you can employ to maximize your performance.

First, as stated before, get a good night's sleep the night before the test (and for several nights before that, if possible). Go into the test with a fresh, alert mind rather than staying up late to study.

Try not to change too much about your normal routine on the day of the test. It's important to eat a nutritious breakfast, but if you normally don't eat breakfast at all, consider eating just a protein bar. If you're a coffee drinker, go ahead and have your normal coffee. Just make sure you time it so that the caffeine doesn't wear off right in the middle of your test. Avoid sugary beverages, and drink enough water to stay hydrated but not so much that you need a restroom break 10 minutes into the test. If your test isn't first thing in the morning, consider going for a walk or doing a light workout before the test to get your blood flowing.

Allow yourself enough time to get ready, and leave for the test with plenty of time to spare so you won't have the anxiety of scrambling to arrive in time. Another reason to be early is to select a good seat. It's helpful to sit away from doors and windows, which can be distracting. Find a good seat, get out your supplies, and settle your mind before the test begins.

When the test begins, start by going over the instructions carefully, even if you already know what to expect. Make sure you avoid any careless mistakes by following the directions.

Then begin working through the questions, pacing yourself as you've practiced. If you're not sure on an answer, don't spend too much time on it, and don't let it shake your confidence. Either skip it and come back later, or eliminate as many wrong answers as possible and guess among the remaining ones. Don't dwell on these questions as you continue—put them out of your mind and focus on what lies ahead.

Be sure to read all of the answer choices, even if you're sure the first one is the right answer. Sometimes you'll find a better one if you keep reading. But don't second-guess yourself if you do immediately know the answer. Your gut instinct is usually right. Don't let test anxiety rob you of the information you know.

If you have time at the end of the test (and if the test format allows), go back and review your answers. Be cautious about changing any, since your first instinct tends to be correct, but make sure you didn't misread any of the questions or accidentally mark the wrong answer choice. Look over any you skipped and make an educated guess.

At the end, leave the test feeling confident. You've done your best, so don't waste time worrying about your performance or wishing you could change anything. Instead, celebrate the successful completion of this test. And finally, use this test to learn how to deal with anxiety even better next time.

> **Review Video: 5 Tips to Beat Test Anxiety**
> Visit mometrix.com/academy and enter code: 570656

Important Qualification

Not all anxiety is created equal. If your test anxiety is causing major issues in your life beyond the classroom or testing center, or if you are experiencing troubling physical symptoms related to your anxiety, it may be a sign of a serious physiological or psychological condition. If this sounds like your situation, we strongly encourage you to seek professional help.

Thank You

We at Mometrix would like to extend our heartfelt thanks to you, our friend and patron, for allowing us to play a part in your journey. It is a privilege to serve people from all walks of life who are unified in their commitment to building the best future they can for themselves.

The preparation you devote to these important testing milestones may be the most valuable educational opportunity you have for making a real difference in your life. We encourage you to put your heart into it—that feeling of succeeding, overcoming, and yes, conquering will be well worth the hours you've invested.

We want to hear your story, your struggles and your successes, and if you see any opportunities for us to improve our materials so we can help others even more effectively in the future, please share that with us as well. **The team at Mometrix would be absolutely thrilled to hear from you!** So please, send us an email (support@mometrix.com) and let's stay in touch.

> **If you'd like some additional help, check out these other resources we offer for your exam:**
> http://mometrixflashcards.com/MLS

Additional Bonus Material

Due to our efforts to try to keep this book to a manageable length, we've created a link that will give you access to all of your additional bonus material.

> **Please visit https://www.mometrix.com/bonus948/mls to access the information.**